MW01165852

CONTENTS

INTRODUCTION 6

CHAPTER 1 BREAKFASTS 8

1. Spinach and Bacon Roll-Ups 8
2. All-in-One Toast 8
3. .Simple Banana and Oat Bread Pudding 8
4. Hash Brown Casserole 9
5. Buttermilk Biscuits 9
6. Ham Hash Brown Cups 9
7. Cheesy Tater Tot Casserole 9
8. Fast Cheesy Broccoli Quiche 10
9. Easy Egg Florentine 10
10. Easy Cheesy Fried Grits 11
11. Shrimp, Spinach and Rice Frittata 11
12. Banana Bread Pudding 11
13. Chicken Breast with Apple 11
14. Easy Western Omelet 12
15. .Asparagus Strata 12
16. Artichoke and Mushroom Frittata 12
17. French Toast Sticks with Strawberry Sauce 13
18. Bacon, Egg and Cheese Breakfast Hash 13

CHAPTER 2 FISH AND SEAFOOD 14

19. Asian Swordfish Steaks 14
20. Crispy Halibut Fillets 14
21. .Salmon Fillet with Tomatoes 14
22. Teriyaki Salmon with Bok Choy 15
23. Golden Fish Fillets 15
24. Tuna, Pineapple, and Grape Kebabs 15
25. Salmon Fillets with Asparagus 16
26. Golden Tuna Lettuce Wraps 16
27. Tilapia Tacos 16
28. Cauliflower and Sole Fritters 17
29. Crispy Salmon Spring Rolls 17
30. Spiced Red Snapper Fillet 17
31. .Fruity Sweet-Sour Snapper Fillet 18
32. Gold Salmon Patties 18
33. Toasted Salmon with Asparagus 18
34. Sheet Pan Shrimp Fajitas 19
35. Cod Fillets 19
36. Baked Cajun Cod 19
37. Crispy Salmon Patties 19
38. Tuna Casserole 20
39. Garlic-Butter Shrimpwith Potatoes 20
40. Easy Salmon Patties 21
41. Broiled Crab Cakes With Herb Sauce 21
42. .Lemon-Honey Snapper with Fruit 21

43. Asian-Inspired Swordfish Steaks 21
44. Baked Sole with Asparagus 22
45. Butter-Wine Baked Salmon 22
46. Broiled Chipotle Tilapia 22
47. Golden Beer-Battered Cod 23
48. Garlicky Cod Fillets 23
49. Dijon Salmon with Green Beans 23
50. Lemony Gold Sole 23
51. .Spicy Shrimp 24
52. Pecan-Crusted Catfish 24
53. Tilapia Meunière 24
54. Garlicky Parmesan-Crusted Hake Fillet 25
55. Fish and Chips 25
56. Air-Fryer Scallops with Lemon-Herb Sauce 25
57. Air Fryer Mahi Mahi with Brown Butter 26
58. Mustard Crusted Salmon 26
59. Cheesy Shrimp 26
60. Hoisin Tuna with Jasmine Rice 26
61. .Golden Fish Sticks 27
62. Panko-Crusted Fish Sticks 27
63. Southern Salmon Bowl 27
64. Panko-Crusted Calamari with Lemon 27
65. Lemony Shrimp with Parsley 28
66. Fast Bacon-Wrapped Scallops 28
67. Panko-Crusted Catfish Nuggets 28
68. Lemony Tilapia Fillet 29
69. .Coconut Spicy Fish 29
70. Lemony Parsley Shrimp 29
71. Toasted Nicoise Salad 29
72. Shrimp Saladwith Caesar Dressing 30
73. Tuna Patties with Cheese Sauced 30
74. .Cheesy Cajun Catfish Cakes 31
75. Garlicky Orange Shrimp 31
76. Easy Coconut Scallops 31
77. Breaded Crab Sticks with Mayo Sauce 32
78. Butter-Wine Baked Salmon Steak 32
79. Shrimp Spring Rolls 32

CHAPTER 3 MAINS 34

80. Marinara Sauce 34
81. Spicy Southwest Seasoning 34
82. .Classic Caesar Salad Dressing 34
83. Baked White Rice 34
84. Beef & Asparagus 34
85. Teriyaki Sauce 35
86. Roast Beef 35

CHAPTER 4 MEATS **36**
87. Easy Spicy Steaks with Salad....................................36
88. Spring Rolls..36
89. Bacon & Broccoli Rice Bowl....................................36
90. Paprika Pork Chops with Corn................................37
91. Chuck Steak and Pork Sausage Meatloaf.............37
92. Barbecue Pork Tenderloin..37
93. Garlic Pork Chops with Roasted Broccoli 37
94. Pork Belly Bites...38
95. Salt-and-Pepper Beef Roast.....................................38
96. Parmesan Pork Chops..38
97. Pork and Beef Stuffed Bell Peppers.....................38
98. Mustard Herbed Pork Chops....................................39
99. Pork Chops with Creamy Dip 39
100. Perfect Air Fryer Pork Chops 40
101. Perfect Rump Roast..40
102. Air Fryer Juicy Steak Fasteat 40
103. Air Fryer Jerk Steak with Compound Butter... 41
104. Air Fryer Bacon Wrapped Beef Tenderloin.....41
105. Slow Roasted Beef Short Ribs 41
106. Air Fryer BBQ Pork Tenderloin............................41
107. Air Fried Masala Chops 42
108. London Broil Steak 42
109. Air Fryer Marinated Steak 42
110. Air Fryer Pork Belly Bites 43
111. Breaded Boneless Pork Chops with Creamy
Dipping Sauce 43
112. Simple Lamb Chops with Horseradish Sauce . 44
113. Easy Cinnamon Steak..44
114. Air Fryer Carne Asada Recipe 44
115. Panko-Crusted Lemony Schnitz e......................45
116. Pork, Bell Pepper, and Pineapple Kebabs 45
117. Fast Salsa Meatballs 46
118. Smoked Paprika Pork and Vegetable Kabobs. 46
119. Fast Bacon-Wrapped Hot Dogs............................46
120. Tangy Pork Ribs 47
121. .Breaded Calf's Liver Strips 47
122. .Golden Pork Tenderloin 47
123. .North African Lamb Kofta......................................47
124. Panko-Crusted Wasabi Spam 48
125. Golden Asparagus and Prosciutto Tart 48
126. Pork Butt with Garlicky Sauce...............................49
127. Apple-Glazed Pork Chops 49
128. Turkish Spicy Lamb Pizza.......................................49
129. Panko-Crusted Beef Meatballs...............................50
130. Cheesy Tomato Sauce Meatloaf............................50
131. Pork, Squash, and Pepper Kebabs 50

132. Ritzy Steak with Mushroom Gravy.....................51
133. Macadamia Nuts Breaded Pork Rack 51
CHAPTER 5 POULTRY **53**
134. Easy Meatballs with Dijon Sauce........................53
135. Easy Air Fryer Grilled Chicken..............................53
136. Chicken Thighs with Rosemary 53
137. Air Fryer Lemon Pepper Chicken 53
138. Air Fryer Chicken Tenders 54
139. Air Fryer General Tso's Chicken Recipe............54
140. Herb Roasted Turkey Breast 54
141. Air Fryer Copycat Chicken Sandwich.................55
142. Sheet Pan Shakshuka 55
143. Quick and Easy Air Fryer BBQ Chicken Wings56
144. Air Fryer Whole Chicken 56
145. Air Fryer Chicken Nuggets......................................56
146. Air Fryer Chicken Teriyaki Bowls.........................57
147. Air Fryer BBQ Drumsticks 57
148. Chicken Curry Salad 58
CHAPTER 6 VEGAN AND VEGETARIAN **59**
149. Onion Rings 59
150. Cauliflower Bites...59
151. Balsamic Asparagus Spears......................................59
152. Baked Potatoes..59
153. Cheesy Egg Rolls 60
154. Vegetarian Pizza 60
155. Brussels Sprout Chips 60
156. Golden Eggplant Slices with Parsley....................60
157. Toasted-Baked Tofu cubes 61
158. Veggie Rolls..61
159. Toasted Vegetables with Rice and Eggs 61
160. Lemony Brussels Sprouts...62
161. Zucchini Lasagna 62
162. Eggplant Pizza...62
163. Cheesy Stuffed Mushrooms with Veggies.........63
164. Toasted Mushrooms, Pepper and Squash 63
165. Fast Lemony Wax Beans...63
166. Sriracha Roasted Potatoes.......................................63
CHAPTER 7 VEGETABLE SIDES **64**
167. Garlicky-Balsamic Asparagus 64
168. Cheesy Buttered Broccoli...64
169. Broccoli with Hot Sauce...64
170. Crispy Brussels Sprouts with Sage.......................64
CHAPTER 8 APPETIZERS AND SNACKS **65**
171. Cheesy Pepperoni Pizza Bites 65
172. Crispy Kale Chips 65
173. Golden Cornmeal Batter Ball 65
174. Bacon Onion Rings...66

175. .Cinnamon Apple Wedges with Yogurt............ 66
176. Hot Corn Tortilla Chips................................ 66
177. Cheesy Jalapeño Peppers............................ 66
178. Crunchy Cod Fingers................................... 67
179. Crispy Cheesy Mixed Snack......................... 67
180. .Crispy Cheesy Zucchini Tots....................... 67
181. Cheesy BBQ Chicken Pizza.......................... 68
182. Crispy Carrot Chips.................................... 68
183. Crispy Apple Chips..................................... 68

CHAPTER 9 DESSERTS...69
184. Easy Vanilla Walnuts Tart........................... 69
185. Golden Bananaswith Chocolate Sauce............. 69
186. Honey Apple-Peach Crumble......................... 69
187. Baked Berries with Coconut Chip.................... 69
188. Simple Blackberry Chocolate Cake 70
189. Caramelized Fruit Skewers 70
190. Vanilla Chocolate Cookies........................... 70
191. .Fast Chocolate Cheesecake......................... 71
192. Peach and Blueberry Tart............................ 71
193. Berries with Nuts Streusel Topping 71
194. Golden Peach and Blueberry Galette................ 72
195. .Coffee Cake... 72
196. Apple and Peach Crisp................................ 73
197. Cacio e Pepe Air-Fried Ravioli...................... 73
198. Easy Chocolate and Coconut Cake.................. 73
199. Chocolate-Coconut Cake.............................. 74
200. Classic Vanilla Pound Cake.......................... 74

**CHAPTER 10 CASSEROLES, FRITTATA, AND
QUICHE 75**
201. Cheesy Chicken Divan................................. 75
202. Cheesy-Creamy Broccoli Casserole................. 75
203. Cheesy Chorizo, Corn, and Potato Frittata....... 75
204. Taco Beef and Green Chile Casserole.............. 75
205. .Golden Asparagus Frittata.......................... 76
206. .Corn and Bell Pepper Casserole 76
207. .Creamy-Mustard Pork Gratin....................... 76
208. .Broccoli, Carrot, and Tomato Quiche............. 77
209. Herbed Cheddar Cheese Frittata.................... 77
210. Cauliflower, Okra, and Pepper Casserole 77
211. Sumptuous Chicken and Vegetable Casserole 78
212. Easy Chickpea and Spinach Casserole 78
213. Classic Mediterranean Quiche 78
214. Cheesy Mushrooms and Spinach Frittata........ 79
215. .Cheesy Asparagus and Grits Casserole........... 79
216. Cauliflower Florets and Pumpkin Casserole... 79
217. .Cheesy-Creamy Green Bean Casserole............ 80

CHAPTER 11 WRAPS AND SANDWICHES.............81

218. .Crunchy Chicken Egg Rolls......................... 81
219. .Panko-Crusted Avocado and Slaw Tacos......... 81
220. Golden Baja Fish Tacos 81
221. Golden Cabbage and Mushroom Spring Rolls 82
222. Cheesy Philly Steaks.................................. 82
223. Cheesy Chicken Wraps................................ 83
224. Golden Avocado and Tomato Egg Rolls............ 83
225. Korean Beef and Onion Tacos 84
226. .Crispy Pea and Potato Samosas................... 84
227. .Cheesy Sweet Potato and Bean Burritos.......... 85
228. Golden Chicken and Yogurt Taquitos.............. 85
229. Turkey Patties with Chive Mayo 85
230. Crunchy Shrimp and Zucchini Potstickers....... 86
231. Cod Tacos with Salsa.................................. 86
232. Golden Spring Rolls 87
233. Creamy-Cheesy Wontons............................ 87
234. Golden Chicken Empanadas......................... 87
235. .Fast Cheesy Bacon and Egg Wraps................ 88
236. Beef and Seeds Burgers.............................. 88
237. Thai Pork Burgers 89

CHAPTER 12 HOLIDAY SPECIALS........................... 90
238. Crispy Arancini.. 90
239. .Fast Banana Cake..................................... 90
240. Sausage Rolls.. 90
241. Blistered Cherry Tomatoes 91
242. Fast Golden Nuggets.................................. 91
243. .Golden Kale Salad Sushi Rolls 91
244. Golden Chocolate and Coconut Macaroons 92
245. Milk-Butter Pecan Tart.............................. 92
246. Cheese Bread (Pão de Queijo)..................... 93
247. Golden Garlicky Olive Stromboli 93
248. Simple Chocolate Buttermilk Cake................. 93
249. Chocolate-Glazed Custard Donut Holes 94
250. Easy Butter Cake...................................... 94
251. Golden Jewish Blintzes............................... 95
252. .Fast Teriyaki Shrimp Skewers...................... 95
253. .Cream Glazed Cinnamon Rolls..................... 96

**CHAPTER 13 FAST AND EASY EVERYDAY
FAVORITES 97**
254. .Fast Traditional Latkes 97
255. Simple Garlicky-Cheesy Shrimps 97
256. Fast Baked Cherry Tomatoes 97
257. Easy Air-Fried Edamame............................. 97
258. .Easy Spicy Old Bay Shrimp......................... 98
259. Fast Corn on the Cob 98
260. Golden Worcestershire Poutine 98
261. Sugary Glazed Apple Fritters....................... 99

262. Chessy Jalapeño Cornbread 99
263. .Panko Salmon and Carrot Croquettes.............. 99
264. .Spicy Chicken Wings 100
265. Air-Fried Lemony Shishito Peppers 100
266. Greek Spanakopita...100
267. Crunchy Sweet Cinnamon Chickpeas.............101
268. Air-Fried Squash with Hazelnuts......................101
269. Crispy Citrus Avocado Wedge Fries 101
270. Lemony-Cheesy Pears 101
271. Crunchy Salty Tortilla Chips 102
272. Air-Fried Okra Chips 102
273. Parsnip Fries with Garlicky Yogurt.................102
274. Golden Bacon Pinwheels......................................102
275. Crispy and Beery Onion Rings 103
276. Classic French Fries...103
CHAPTER 14 ROTISSERIE RECIPES 104
277. Lemony Rotisserie Lamb Leg.............................104
278. Roasted Pears 104
279. Chicken Breast with Veggies 104
280. Roasted Spaghetti Squash...................................104
281. Toasted Rotisserie Pork Shoulder....................105

282. Roasted Italian Sausage 105
283. Slow Roasted Herb Chicken 105
284. Apple, Carrot, and Onion Stuffed Turkey 106
285. Spicy-Sweet Pork Tenderloin............................ 106
286. Standing Rib Roast.. 106
287. Simple Air-Fried Beef Roast............................... 106
288. Air-Fried Lemony-Garlicky Chicken............... 107
289. Roasted Vegetable Pasta...................................... 107
290. Air-Fried Whole Chicken 107
291. Honey-Glazed Ham 108
292. Roasted Filet Mignon 108
293. Rotisserie Red Wine Lamb 108
294. Miso Glazed Salmon... 109
295. Toasted Marinated Medium Rare Beef........... 109
CHAPTER 15: BREAD & PIZZA............................110
296. Pizza Toast 110
297. Baked Meatloaf.. 110
298. Strawberry Ricotta Toast.................................... 110
299. Mediterranean Baked Fish 111
300. Baked Cinnamon Apple....................................... 111

INTRODUCTION

What is the PowerXL Air Fryer Grill?

A multifunction air fryer and grill, the PowerXL Air Fryer Grill offers a plethora of menu possibilities with up to 70 percent fewer calories from fat than traditional frying.

It features eight cooking presets that let you air fry and grill at the same time, air fry, grill, bake, toast, broil, rotisserie or reheat food with less cooking oil or none at all. It also does not require thawing and can cook food straight from the freezer.

The PowerXL Air Fryer Grill boasts an up to 450-degree superheated air circulation that ensures the food is cooked evenly on all sides, extra crispy on the outside and tenderly juicy on the inside.

The unit heats almost instantly with a smart preheat feature that starts the timer only when it reaches the desired temperature. It also shuts off automatically.

Equipped with two racks, the PowerXL Air Fryer Grill can cook as much as 4.5 times more food than traditionally smaller air fryers. Ideal for cooking meals for the whole family or when hosting a gathering, the large capacity allows the unit to accommodate up to 10 pounds of chicken, a 12-inch round pizza, six toast slices or bagels, or the equivalent load of a 4.5-quart Dutch oven.

How Does it Work?

In general, air fryers feature a fan that circulates hot air within its chambers in order to cook food. The hot air radiates from the chamber through the heating elements near the food.

To control the temperature, excess hot air is released through an air inlet on the top and an exhaust at the back of the unit.

Instead of being completely submerged in hot oil, food in air fryers are air-heated to induce the Maillard reaction, resulting in browned food with a distinct aroma and taste.

The PowerXL Air Fryer Grill's fan is equipped with turbo blades that are more powerful than its competitors. These blades are angled strategically in order to distribute heat evenly over the surface of the food. Depending on the kind of food, cooking times are reduced by at least 20 percent in comparison with that of traditional ovens.

It also comes with a non-stick grill plate that creates gorgeous grill marks and chargrill flavor without the use of charcoal or propane

Steps to Using the PowerXL Air Fryer Grill

Operating your PowerXL Air Fryer Grill is a breeze with its easy to assemble parts and accessories and simple control panel. After choosing the desired settings, you can just leave it and forget about it until it is time to eat.

Before using the unit for the first time, read all materials, labels and stickers. Remove all packaging, labels and stickers prior to operation. Hand wash all removable parts and accessories with soapy water.

Place the PowerXL Air Fryer Grill on a safe, stable, level, horizontal and heat-resistant surface in an area with good air circulation. Keep the unit away from hot surfaces, other objects or appliances, and combustible materials. It is advisable to plug the unit to a designated outlet.

Carefully assemble the parts and accessories. On the left side of the air fryer's door, you will see guides that indicate the ideal place for the racks and pans. The drip tray should be kept below the heating elements at all times when cooking.

Preheat the unit to allow the manufacturer's protective coating to burn, and then wipe off with a warm moist cloth.

Lightly grease the food before cooking to ensure that it would not stick to the pan or to each other. You may opt to use healthier plant-based oils like avocado and olive. If you are cooking wet food such as marinated meat, pat them dry first to avoid excessive splattering and smoke while cooking.

Avoid overcrowding the food for hot air to circulate effectively and achieve crispy results. Also keep in mind that air fryers cook food faster so follow recommended temperature settings to avoid overcooking or burning.

There are three knobs for: (1) adjusting temperature (up to 450 degrees) and toast darkness options, (2) selecting cooking function (air fry, air fry/grill, grill, broil, pizza/bake, reheat, toast/bagel, rotisserie), and setting the timer (up to 120 minutes).

To make toast, set the toast darkness first and then choose the toast/bagel function. Next, turn the timer knob clockwise past the 20-minute mark, and then rotate counterclockwise to the toast icon.

For the rest of the cooking functions, turn the timer knob past the 20-minute mark before adjusting it to the desired time.

You must select a cooking function for the device to start. When a cooking function and time have been set, the light will turn on. Once the timer expires, the light goes off.

Benefits of the PowerXL Air Fryer Grill

Authentic BBQ Flavors & Char Grill Marks

The same juicy grill marks and delicious char grilled flavors of an outdoor BBQ are provided by the high density nonstick grill plate with raised ridges. It does not require propane or charcoal.

7x More Flow of Superheated Air

In a whirlwind of superheated hot air rather than fat, grill and air fried your favorite meals crisply. Intuitive heating combined with high-speed seamless air flow helps minimize cooking time for juicier, more uniformly cooked, crispier results. Grilled steaks on nonstick grill pans with grill marks

Tips for Care & Maintenance

It is a good practice to visually inspect your PowerXL Air Fryer before each use to make sure that it will function safely and properly. Air fryers may be built to last a long time but just like any other kitchen appliance, you may encounter a few minor and easy-to-fix problems with them from time to time.

Cleaning & Deodorizing

Make sure that the unit is clean before each use. Check the inside for any debris or accumulated dust if you have not been using your unit for some time.

Clean the unit immediately after each use, especially after cooking foods with a pungent smell. Unplug the air fryer and allow it to cool down for at least 30 minutes.

All of the removable parts and accessories are dishwasher safe. If you prefer to handwash, use a mild detergent and soft moist cloth. Do not use abrasive cleaning materials.

Regularly empty the accumulated fat from the bottom of the machine to avoid excessive smoke when cooking.

Storage

After cleaning, make sure that the unit and all its parts and components are dry before storing away. Ensure that the unit will be kept in a stable, level and upright position while in storage. Keep it in a cool, dry place.

Special tips to use the PowerXL Air Fryer Grill

Use Oven Mitts, Utensils

After a cooking cycle is completed, you can expect the accessories inside to be hot when you open up your PowerXL Air Fryer Grill. Therefore, when sticking your hands inside the device, you should wear oven mitts, and it's also best to use cooking utensils instead of your hands to remove the food. Similarly, you can let it cool down for at least a half-hour while the appliance is switched off before removing any attachments to move it to your dishwasher or sink.

CHAPTER 1 BREAKFASTS

1.   Spinach and Bacon Roll-Ups

Prep time: 5 minutes | Cook time: 8 to 9 minutes | Serves 4

4 flour tortillas (6- or 7-inch size)
4 slices Swiss cheese
1 cup baby spinach leaves
4 slices turkey bacon

Special Equipment:

4 toothpicks, soak in water for at least 30 minutes

1.   On a clean work surface, top each tortilla with one slice of cheese and ¼ cup of spinach, then tightly roll them up.

2.   Wrap each tortilla with a strip of turkey bacon and secure with a toothpick.

3.   Arrange the roll-ups in the air fryer basket, leaving space between each roll-up.

4.   Place the basket on the air fry position. Select Air Fry, set temperature to 390ºF (199ºC), and set time to 8 minutes.

5.   After 4 minutes, remove the basket from the air fryer grill. Flip the roll-ups with tongs and rearrange them for more even cooking. Return to the air fryer grill and continue cooking for another 4 minutes.

6.   When cooking is complete, the bacon should be crisp. If necessary, continue cooking for 1 minute more. Remove the basket from the air fryer grill. Rest for 5 minutes and remove the toothpicks before serving.

2.   All-in-One Toast

Prep time: 5 minutes | Cook time: 6 minutes | Serves: 1

1 slice bread
1 teaspoon butter, at room temperature
1 egg
Salt and freshly ground black pepper, to taste
2 teaspoons diced ham
1 tablespoon grated Cheddar cheese

1.   On a clean work surface, use a 2½-inch biscuit cutter to make a hole in the center of the bread slice with about ½-inch of bread remaining.

2.   Spread the butter on both sides of the bread slice. Crack the egg into the hole and season with salt and pepper to taste. Transfer the bread to the air fryer basket.

3.   Place the basket on the air fry position. Select Air Fry, set temperature to 325ºF (163ºC), and set time to 6 minutes.

4.   After 5 minutes, remove the basket from the air fryer grill. Scatter the cheese and diced ham on top and continue cooking for an additional 1 minute.

5.   When cooking is complete, the egg should be set and the cheese should be melted. Remove the toast from the air fryer grill to a plate and let cool for 5 minutes before serving.

3.   .Simple Banana and Oat Bread Pudding

Prep time: 10 minutes | Cook time: 16 minutes | Serves 4

2 medium ripe bananas, mashed
½ cup low-fat milk
2 tablespoons peanut butter
2 tablespoons maple syrup
1 teaspoon vanilla extract
1 teaspoon ground cinnamon
2 slices whole-grain bread, cut into bite-sized cubes
¼ cup quick oats
Cooking spray

1.   Spritz a baking dish lightly with cooking spray.

2.   Mix the bananas, milk, peanut butter, maple syrup, vanilla, and cinnamon in a large mixing bowl and stir until well incorporated.

3.   Add the bread cubes to the banana mixture and stir until thoroughly coated. Fold in the oats and stir to combine.

4.   Transfer the mixture to the baking dish. Wrap the baking dish in aluminum foil.

5.   Place the baking dish on the air fry position.

6.   Select Air Fry, set temperature to 350ºF (180ºC) and set time to 16 minutes.

7. After 10 minutes, remove the baking dish from the air fryer grill. Remove the foil. Return the baking dish to the air fryer grill and continue to cook another 6 minutes.

8. When done, the pudding should be set.

9. Let the pudding cool for 5 minutes before serving.

4. Hash Brown Casserole

Prep time: 15 minutes | Cook time: 30 minutes | Serves 4

3½ cups frozen hash browns, thawed
1 teaspoon salt
1 teaspoon freshly ground black pepper
1 (10.5-ounce / 298-g) can cream of chicken soup
3 tablespoons butter, melted
½ cup sour cream
1 cup minced onion
½ cup shredded sharp Cheddar cheese
Cooking spray

1. Put the hash browns in a large bowl and season with salt and black pepper. Add the cream of chicken soup, melted butter, and sour cream and stir until well incorporated. Mix in the minced onion and cheese and stir well.

2. Spray a baking pan with cooking spray.

3. Spread the hash brown mixture evenly into the baking pan.

4. Place the pan on the bake position.

5. Select Bake, set temperature to 325ºF (163ºC) and set time to 30 minutes.

6. When cooked, the hash brown mixture will be browned.

7. Cool for 5 minutes before serving.

5. Buttermilk Biscuits

Prep time: 5 minutes | Cook time: 18 minutes | Makes 16 biscuits

2½ cups all-purpose flour
1 tablespoon baking powder
1 teaspoon kosher salt
1 teaspoon sugar
½ teaspoon baking soda
1 cup buttermilk, chilled
8 tablespoons (1 stick) unsalted butter, at room temperature

1. Stir together the flour, baking powder, salt, sugar, and baking powder in a large bowl.

2. Add the butter and stir to mix well. Pour in the buttermilk and stir with a rubber spatula just until incorporated.

3. Place the dough onto a lightly floured surface and roll the dough out to a disk, ½ inch thick. Cut out the biscuits with a 2-inch round cutter and re-roll any scraps until you have 16 biscuits.

4. Arrange the biscuits in the air fryer basket in a single layer.

5. Place the basket on the bake position.

6. Select Bake, set temperature to 325ºF (163ºC), and set time to 18 minutes.

7. When cooked, the biscuits will be golden brown.

8. Remove from the air fryer grill to a plate and serve hot.

6. Ham Hash Brown Cups

Prep time: 10 minutes | Cook time: 9 minutes | Serves 6

4 eggs, beaten
1 cup diced ham
2¼ cups frozen hash browns, thawed
½ cup shredded Cheddar cheese
½ teaspoon Cajun seasoning
Cooking spray

1. Lightly spritz a 12-cup muffin tin with cooking spray.

2. Combine the beaten eggs, diced ham, hash browns, cheese, and Cajun seasoning in a medium bowl and stir until well blended.

3. Spoon a heaping 1½ tablespoons of egg mixture into each muffin cup.

4. Place the muffin tin on the bake position.

5. Select Bake, set temperature to 350ºF (180ºC) and set time to 9 minutes.

6. When cooked, the muffins will be golden brown.

7. Allow to cool for 5 to 10 minutes on a wire rack and serve warm.

7. Cheesy Tater Tot Casserole

Prep time: 5 minutes | Cook time: 17 to 18 minutes | Serves 4

4 eggs

1 cup milk
Salt and pepper, to taste
Cooking spray
12 ounces (340 g) ground chicken sausage
1 pound (454 g) frozen tater tots, thawed
¾ cup grated Cheddar cheese

1.   Whisk together the eggs and milk in a medium bowl. Season with salt and pepper to taste and stir until mixed. Set aside.

2.   Place a skillet over medium-high heat and spritz with cooking spray. Place the ground sausage in the skillet and break it into smaller pieces with a spatula or spoon. Cook for 3 to 4 minutes until the sausage Starts to brown, stirring occasionally. Remove from heat and set aside.

3.   Coat a baking pan with cooking spray. Arrange the tater tots in the baking pan.

4.   Place the pan on the bake position.

5.   Select Bake, set temperature to 400ºF (205ºC) and set time to 14 minutes.

6.   After 6 minutes, remove the pan from the air fryer grill. Stir the tater tots and add the egg mixture and cooked sausage. Return the pan to the air fryer grill and continue cooking.

7.   After another 6 minutes, remove the pan from the air fryer grill. Scatter the cheese on top of the tater tots. Return the pan to the air fryer grill and continue to cook for 2 minutes more.

8.   When done, the cheese should be bubbly and melted.

9.   Let the mixture cool for 5 minutes and serve warm.

8.   Fast Cheesy Broccoli Quiche

Prep time: 5 minutes | Cook time: 10 minutes | Serves 4

Cooking spray
1 cup broccoli florets
¾ cup chopped Toasted red peppers
1¼ cups grated Fontina cheese
6 eggs
¾ cup heavy cream
½ teaspoon salt
Freshly ground black pepper, to taste

1.   Spritz a baking pan with cooking spray

2.   Add the broccoli florets and Toasted red peppers to the pan and scatter the grated Fontina cheese on top.

3.   In a bowl, beat together the eggs and heavy cream. Sprinkle with salt and pepper. Pour the egg mixture over the top of the cheese. Wrap the pan in foil.

4.   Place the pan on the air fry position.

5.   Select Air Fry, set temperature to 325ºF (163ºC) and set time to 10 minutes.

6.   After 8 minutes, remove the pan from the air fryer grill. Remove the foil. Return the pan to the air fryer grill and continue to cook another 2 minutes.

7.   When cooked, the quiche should be golden brown.

8.   Rest for 5 minutes before cutting into wedges and serve warm.

9.   Easy Egg Florentine

Prep time: 10 minutes | Cook time: 15 minutes | Serves 4

3 cups frozen spinach, thawed and drained
2 tablespoons heavy cream
¼ teaspoon kosher salt
⅛ teaspoon freshly ground black pepper
2 garlic cloves, minced
4 ounces (113 g) Ricotta cheese
½ cup panko bread crumbs
3 tablespoons grated Parmesan cheese
2 teaspoons unsalted butter, melted
4 large eggs

1.   In a medium bowl, whisk together the spinach, heavy cream, salt, pepper, garlic and Ricotta cheese.

2.   In a small bowl, whisk together the bread crumbs, Parmesan cheese and butter. Set aside.

3.   Spoon the spinach mixture on the sheet pan and form four even circles.

4.   Place the pan on the toast position.

5.   Select Toast, set temperature to 375ºF (190ºC) and set time to 15 minutes.

6.   After 8 minutes, remove the pan from the air fryer grill. The spinach should be bubbling. With the back of a large spoon, make indentations in the spinach for the eggs. Crack the eggs into the indentations and sprinkle the panko mixture over the

surface of the eggs. Return the pan to the air fryer grill to continue cooking.

7.   When cooking is complete, remove the pan from the air fryer grill. Serve hot.

10. Easy Cheesy Fried Grits

Prep time: 10 minutes | Cook time: 11 minutes | Serves 4

$^2/_3$ cup instant grits
1 teaspoon salt
1 teaspoon freshly ground black pepper
3 ounces (85 g) cream cheese, at room temperature
¾ cup whole or 2% milk
1 large egg, beaten
1 tablespoon butter, melted
1 cup shredded mild Cheddar cheese
Cooking spray

1.   Mix the grits, salt, and black pepper in a large bowl. Add the cream cheese, milk, beaten egg, and melted butter and whisk to combine. Fold in the Cheddar cheese and stir well.
2.   Spray a baking pan with cooking spray. Spread the grits mixture into the baking pan.
3.   Place the pan on the air fry position.
4.   Select Air Fry, set temperature to 400ºF (205ºC) and set time to 11 minutes. Stir the mixture halfway through the cooking time.
5.   When done, a knife inserted in the center should come out clean.
6.   Rest for 5 minutes and serve warm.

11. Shrimp, Spinach and Rice Frittata

Prep time: 15 minutes | Cook time: 16 minutes | Serves 4

4 eggs
Pinch salt
½ cup cooked rice
½ cup baby spinach
½ cup chopped cooked shrimp
½ cup grated Monterey Jack cheese
Nonstick cooking spray

1.   Spritz a baking pan with nonstick cooking spray.
2.   Whisk the eggs and salt in a small bowl until frothy.

3.   Place the cooked rice, baby spinach, and shrimp in the baking pan. Pour in the whisked eggs and scatter the cheese on top.
4.   Place the pan on the bake position.
5.   Select Bake, set temperature to 320ºF (160ºC) and set time to 16 minutes.
6.   When cooking is complete, the frittata should be golden and puffy.
7.   Let the frittata cool for 5 minutes before slicing to serve.

12. Banana Bread Pudding

Prep time: 10 minutes | Cook time: 18 minutes | Serves 4

2 medium ripe bananas, mashed
½ cup low-fat milk
2 tablespoons maple syrup
2 tablespoons peanut butter
1 teaspoon vanilla extract
1 teaspoon ground cinnamon
2 slices whole-grain bread, torn into bite-sized pieces
¼ cup quick oats
Cooking spray

1.   Spritz the sheet pan with cooking spray.
2.   In a large bowl, combine the bananas, maple syrup, peanut butter, milk, vanilla extract and cinnamon. Use an immersion blender to mix until well combined.
3.   Stir in the bread pieces to coat well. Add the oats and stir until everything is combined.
4.   Transfer the mixture to the sheet pan. Cover with the aluminum foil.
5.   Place the pan on the air fry position.
6.   Select Air Fry, set temperature to 375ºF (190ºC) and set time to 18 minutes.
7.   After 10 minutes, remove the foil and continue to cook for 8 minutes.
8.   Serve immediately.

13. Chicken Breast with Apple

Prep time: 15 minutes | Cook time: 10 minutes | Makes 8 patties

1 egg white
2 garlic cloves, minced
1 Granny Smith apple, peeled and finely chopped
$^1/_3$ cup minced onion
3 tablespoons ground almonds

2 tablespoons apple juice

⅛ teaspoon freshly ground black pepper

1 pound (454 g) ground chicken breast

1. Combine all the ingredients except the chicken in a medium mixing bowl and stir well.

2. Add the chicken breast to the apple mixture and mix with your hands until well incorporated.

3. Divide the mixture into 8 equal portions and shape into patties. Arrange the patties in the air fry basket.

4. Place the air fry basket on the air fry position.

5. Select Air Fry, set temperature to 330ºF (166ºC) and set time to 10 minutes.

6. When done, a meat thermometer inserted in the center of the chicken should reach at least 165ºF (74ºC).

7. Remove from the air fryer grill to a plate. Let the chicken cool for 5 minutes and serve warm.

14. Easy Western Omelet

Prep time: 5 minutes | Cook time: 20 minutes | Serves 2

¼ cup chopped bell pepper, green or red

¼ cup chopped onion

¼ cup diced ham

1 teaspoon butter

4 large eggs

⅛ teaspoon salt

2 tablespoons milk

¾ cup shredded sharp Cheddar cheese

1. Put the bell pepper, onion, ham, and butter in a baking pan and mix well.

2. Place the pan on the air fry position.

3. Select Air Fry, set temperature to 390ºF (199ºC) and set time to 5 minutes.

4. After 1 minute, remove the pan from the air fryer grill. Stir the mixture. Return the pan to the air fryer grill and continue to cook for another 4 minutes.

5. When done, the veggies should be softened.

6. Whisk together the eggs, salt, and milk in a bowl. Pour the egg mixture over the veggie mixture.

7. Place the pan on the bake position.

8. Select Bake, set temperature to 360ºF (182ºC) and set time to 15 minutes.

9. After 14 minutes, remove the pan from the air fryer grill. Scatter the omelet with the shredded

cheese. Return the pan to the air fryer grill and continue to cook for another 1 minute.

10. When cooking is complete, the top will be lightly golden browned, the eggs will be set and the cheese will be melted.

11. Let the omelet cool for 5 minutes before serving.

15. .Asparagus Strata

Prep time: 10 minutes | Cook time: 17 minutes | Serves 4

6 asparagus spears, cut into 2-inch pieces

1 tablespoon water

2 slices whole-wheat bread, cut into ½-inch cubes

4 eggs

3 tablespoons whole milk

½ cup grated Havarti or Swiss cheese

2 tablespoons chopped flat-leaf parsley

Pinch salt

Freshly ground black pepper, to taste

Cooking spray

1. Add the asparagus spears and 1 tablespoon of water in a baking pan.

2. Place the pan on the bake position.

3. Select Bake, set temperature to 330ºF (166ºC) and set time to 4 minutes.

4. When cooking is complete, the asparagus spears will be crisp-tender.

5. Remove the asparagus from the pan and drain on paper towels.

6. Spritz the pan with cooking spray. Place the bread and asparagus in the pan.

7. Whisk together the eggs and milk in a medium mixing bowl until creamy. Fold in the cheese, parsley, salt, and pepper and stir to combine. Pour this mixture into the baking pan.

8. Select Bake and set time to 13 minutes. Place the pan back to the air fryer grill. When done, the eggs will be set and the top will be lightly browned.

9. Let cool for 5 minutes before slicing and serving.

16. Artichoke and Mushroom Frittata

Prep time: 10 minutes | Cook time: 15 minutes | Serves 6

8 eggs

½ teaspoon kosher salt

¼ cup whole milk

¾ cup shredded Mozzarella cheese, divided

2 tablespoons unsalted butter, melted

¼ cup chopped onion

1 cup coarsely chopped artichoke hearts

½ cup mushrooms

¼ cup grated Parmesan cheese

¼ teaspoon freshly ground black pepper

1. In a medium bowl, whisk together the eggs and salt. Let rest for a minute or two, then pour in the milk and whisk again. Stir in ½ cup of the Mozzarella cheese.

2. Grease the sheet pan with the butter. Stir in the onion and artichoke hearts and toss to coat with the butter.

3. Place the pan on the toast position.

4. Select Toast, set temperature to 375ºF (190ºC) and set time to 12 minutes.

5. After 5 minutes, remove the pan. Spread the mushrooms over the vegetables. Pour the egg mixture on top. Stir gently just to distribute the vegetables evenly. Return the pan to the air fryer grill and continue cooking for 5 to 7 minutes, or until the edges are set. The center will still be quite liquid.

6. Select Broil, set temperature to Low and set time to 3 minutes. Place the pan on the broil position.

7. After 1 minute, remove the pan and sprinkle the remaining ¼ cup of the Mozzarella and Parmesan cheese over the frittata. Return the pan to the air fryer grill and continue cooking for 2 minutes.

8. When cooking is complete, the cheese should be melted with the top completely set but not browned. Sprinkle the black pepper on top and serve.

17. French Toast Sticks with Strawberry Sauce

Prep time: 5 minutes | Cook time: 12 minutes | Serves 4

3 slices low-sodium whole-wheat bread, each cut into 4 strips

1 tablespoon unsalted butter, melted

1 tablespoon sugar

1 tablespoon 2 percent milk

1 egg, beaten

1 egg white

1 cup sliced fresh strawberries

1 tablespoon freshly squeezed lemon juice

1. Arrange the bread strips on a plate and drizzle with the melted butter.

2. In a bowl, whisk together the sugar, milk, egg and egg white.

3. Dredge the bread strips into the egg mixture and place on a wire rack to let the batter drip off. Arrange half the coated bread strips on the sheet pan.

4. Place the pan on the air fry position.

5. Select Air Fry, set temperature to 380ºF (193ºC) and set time to 6 minutes.

6. After 3 minutes, remove the pan from the air fryer grill. Use tongs to turn the strips over. Rotate the pan and return the pan to the air fryer grill to continue cooking.

7. When cooking is complete, the strips should be golden brown.

8. In a small bowl, mash the strawberries with a fork and stir in the lemon juice. Serve the French toast sticks with the strawberry sauce.

18. Bacon, Egg and Cheese Breakfast Hash

There is no better option for breakfast!

Prep time and cooking time: 35 minutes | Serves: 4

Ingredients to Use:

2 slices of bacon

4 tiny potatoes

1/4 tomato

1 egg

1/4 cup of shredded cheese

Step-by-step direction to cook:

1. Preheat the PowerXL Air Fryer Grill to 200ºC or 400ºF on bake mode. Set bits of bacon on a double-layer tin foil.

2. Cut the vegetables to put over the bacon. Crack an egg over it.

3. Shape the tin foil into a bowl and cook it in the PowerXL Air Fryer Grill at 177ºC or 350ºF for 15-20 minutes. Put some shredded cheese on top.

Nutritional Value per Serving:

Calories: 150.5 kcal, Carbs: 18g, Protein: 6g, Fat: 6g.

CHAPTER 2 FISH AND SEAFOOD

19. Asian Swordfish Steaks

Prep time: 10 minutes | Cook time: 8 minutes | Serves 4

4 (4-ounce / 113-g) swordfish steaks
½ teaspoon toasted sesame oil
1 jalapeño pepper, finely minced
2 garlic cloves, grated
2 tablespoons freshly squeezed lemon juice
1 tablespoon grated fresh ginger
½ teaspoon Chinese five-spice powder
⅛ teaspoon freshly ground black pepper

1.   On a clean work surface, place the swordfish steaks and brush both sides of the fish with the sesame oil.
2.   Combine the lemon juice, jalapeño, garlic, ginger, five-spice powder, and black pepper in a small bowl and stir to mix well. Rub the mixture all over the fish until completely coated. Allow to sit for 10 minutes.
3.   When ready, arrange the swordfish steaks in the air fry basket.
4.   Place the basket on the air fry position.
5.   Select Air Fry, set temperature to 380ºF (193ºC), and set time to 8 minutes. Flip the steaks halfway through.
6.   When cooking is complete, remove from the air fryer grill and cool for 5 minutes before serving.

20. Crispy Halibut Fillets

Prep time: 5 minutes | Cook time: 10 minutes | Serves 4

2 medium-sized halibut fillets
Dash of tabasco sauce
1 teaspoon curry powder
½ teaspoon ground coriander
½ teaspoon hot paprika
Kosher salt and freshly cracked mixed peppercorns, to taste
2 eggs
½ cup grated Parmesan cheese
1½ tablespoons olive oil

1.   On a clean work surface, drizzle the halibut fillets with the tabasco sauce. Sprinkle with the curry powder, hot paprika, coriander, salt, and cracked mixed peppercorns. Set aside.
2.   In a shallow bowl, beat the eggs until frothy. In another shallow bowl, combine the Parmesan cheese and olive oil.
3.   One at a time, dredge the halibut fillets in the beaten eggs, shaking off any excess, then roll them over the Parmesan cheese until evenly coated.
4.   Arrange the halibut fillets in the air fry basket in a single layer.
5.   Place the basket on the toast position.
6.   Select Toast, set temperature to 365ºF (185ºC), and set time to 10 minutes.
7.   When cooking is complete, the fish should be golden brown and crisp. Cool for 5 minutes before serving.

21. .Salmon Fillet with Tomatoes

Prep time: 10 minutes | Cook time: 15 minutes | Serves 4

4 (6-ounce / 170-g) salmon fillets, patted dry
1 teaspoon kosher salt, divided
2 pints cherry or grape tomatoes, halved if large, divided
3 tablespoons extra-virgin olive oil, divided
2 garlic cloves, minced
1 small red bell pepper, deseeded and chopped
2 tablespoons chopped fresh basil, divided

1.   Season both sides of the salmon with ½ teaspoon of kosher salt.
2.   Put about half of the tomatoes in a large bowl, along with 2 tablespoons of olive oil, the remaining ½ teaspoon of kosher salt, bell pepper, garlic, and 1 tablespoon of basil. Toss to coat and then transfer to the sheet pan.
3.   Arrange the salmon fillets on the sheet pan, skin-side down. Brush them with the remaining 1 tablespoon of olive oil.
4.   Place the pan on the toast position.
5.   Select Toast, set temperature to 375ºF (190ºC), and set time to 15 minutes.
6.   After 7 minutes, remove the pan and fold in the remaining tomatoes. Return the pan to the air fryer grill and continue cooking.

7.   When cooked, remove the pan from the air fryer grill. Serve sprinkled with the remaining 1 tablespoon of basil.

22. Teriyaki Salmon with Bok Choy

Prep time: 15 minutes | Cook time: 15 minutes | Serves 4

¾ cup Teriyaki sauce , divided
4 (6-ounce / 170-g) skinless salmon fillets
4 heads baby bok choy, root ends trimmed off and cut in half lengthwise through the root
1 teaspoon sesame oil
1 tablespoon vegetable oil
1 tablespoon toasted sesame seeds

1.   Set aside ¼ cup of Teriyaki sauce and pour the remaining sauce into a resealable plastic bag. Put the salmon into the bag and seal, squeezing as much air out as possible. Allow the salmon to marinate for at least 10 minutes.
2.   Arrange the bok choy halves on the sheet pan. Drizzle the oils over the vegetables, tossing to coat. Drizzle about 1 tablespoon of the reserved Teriyaki sauce over the bok choy, then push them to the sides of the sheet pan.
3.   Put the salmon fillets in the middle of the sheet pan.
4.   Place the pan on the toast position.
5.   Select Toast, set temperature to 375ºF (190ºC), and set time to 15 minutes.
6.   When done, remove the pan and brush the salmon with the remaining Teriyaki sauce. Serve garnished with the sesame seeds.

23. Golden Fish Fillets

Prep time: 20 minutes | Cook time: 7 minutes | Serves 4

1 pound (454 g) fish fillets
1 tablespoon coarse brown mustard
1 teaspoon Worcestershire sauce
½ teaspoon hot sauce
Salt, to taste
Cooking spray
Crumb Coating:
¾ cup panko bread crumbs
¼ cup stone-ground cornmeal
¼ teaspoon salt

1.   On your cutting board, cut the fish fillets crosswise into slices, about 1 inch wide.
2.   In a small bowl, stir together the Worcestershire sauce, mustard, and hot sauce to make a paste and rub this paste on all sides of the fillets. Season with salt to taste.
3.   In a shallow bowl, thoroughly combine all the ingredients for the crumb coating and spread them on a sheet of wax paper.
4.   Roll the fish fillets in the crumb mixture until thickly coated. Spritz all sides of the fish with cooking spray, then arrange them in the air fry basket in a single layer.
5.   Place the air fry basket into the air fryer grill.
6.   Select Air Fry, set temperature to 400ºF (205ºC), and set time to 7 minutes.
7.   When cooking is complete, the fish should flake apart with a fork. Remove from the air fryer grill and serve warm.

24. Tuna, Pineapple, and Grape Kebabs

Prep time: 15 minutes | Cook time: 10 minutes | Serves 4
Kebabs:
1 pound (454 g) tuna steaks, cut into 1-inch cubes
½ cup large red grapes
½ cup canned pineapple chunks, drained, juice reserved
Marinade:
1 tablespoon honey
1 teaspoon olive oil
2 teaspoons grated fresh ginger
Pinch cayenne pepper
Special Equipment:
4 metal skewers

1.   Make the kebabs: Thread, alternating tuna cubes, red grapes, and pineapple chunks onto the metal skewers.
2.   Make the marinade: Whisk together the honey, olive oil, ginger, and cayenne pepper in a small bowl. Brush generously the marinade over the kebabs and allow to sit for 10 minutes.
3.   When ready, transfer the kebabs to the air fry basket.
4.   Place the basket on the air fry position.

5. Select Air Fry, set temperature to 370ºF (188ºC), and set time to 10 minutes.

6. After 5 minutes, remove from the air fryer grill and flip the kebabs and brush with the remaining marinade. Return the basket to the air fryer grill and continue cooking for an additional 5 minutes.

7. When cooking is complete, the kebabs should reach an internal temperature of 145ºF (63ºC) on a meat thermometer. Remove from the air fryer grill and discard any remaining marinade. Serve hot.

25. Salmon Fillets with Asparagus

Prep time: 5 minutes | Cook time: 12 minutes | Serves 2

2 teaspoons olive oil, plus additional for drizzling
2 (5-ounce / 142-g) salmon fillets, with skin
Salt and freshly ground black pepper, to taste
1 bunch asparagus, trimmed
1 teaspoon dried tarragon
1 teaspoon dried chives
Fresh lemon wedges, for serving

1. Rub the olive oil all over the salmon fillets. Sprinkle with salt and pepper to taste.

2. Put the asparagus on a foil-lined baking sheet and place the salmon fillets on top, skin-side down.

3. Place the pan on the toast position.

4. Select Toast, set temperature to 425ºF (220ºC), and set time to 12 minutes.

5. When cooked, the fillets should register 145ºF (63ºC) on an instant-read thermometer. Remove from the air fryer grill and cut the salmon fillets in half crosswise, then use a metal spatula to lift flesh from skin and transfer to a serving plate. Discard the skin and drizzle the salmon fillets with additional olive oil. Scatter with the herbs.

6. Serve the salmon fillets with Toasted asparagus spears and lemon wedges on the side.

26. Golden Tuna Lettuce Wraps

Prep time: 10 minutes | Cook time: 4 to 7 minutes | Serves 4

1 pound (454 g) fresh tuna steak, cut into 1-inch cubes
2 garlic cloves, minced
1 tablespoon grated fresh ginger
½ teaspoon toasted sesame oil
4 low-sodium whole-wheat tortillas
2 cups shredded romaine lettuce
1 red bell pepper, thinly sliced
¼ cup low-fat mayonnaise

1. Combine the tuna cubes, ginger, garlic, and sesame oil in a medium bowl and toss until well coated. Allow to sit for 10 minutes.

2. When ready, place the tuna cubes in the air fry basket.

3. Place the basket on the air fry position.

4. Select Air Fry, set temperature to 390ºF (199ºC), and set time to 6 minutes.

5. When cooking is complete, the tuna cubes should be cooked through and golden brown. Remove the tuna cubes from the air fryer grill to a plate.

6. Make the wraps: Place the tortillas on a flat work surface and top each tortilla evenly with the cooked tuna, lettuce, bell pepper, and finish with the mayonnaise. Roll them up and serve immediately.

27. Tilapia Tacos

Prep time: 10 minutes | Cook time: 10 to 15 minutes | Serves 6

1 tablespoon avocado oil
1 tablespoon Cajun seasoning
4 (5 to 6 ounce / 142 to 170 g) tilapia fillets
1 (14-ounce / 397-g) package coleslaw mix
12 corn tortillas
2 limes, cut into wedges

1. Line a baking pan with parchment paper.

2. In a shallow bowl, stir together the avocado oil and Cajun seasoning to make a marinade. Place the tilapia fillets into the bowl, turning to coat evenly.

3. Put the fillets in the baking pan in a single layer.

4. Slide the pan into the air fryer grill.

5. Select Air Fry, set temperature to 375ºF (190ºC), and set time to 10 minutes.

6. When cooked, the fish should be flaky. If necessary, continue cooking for 5 minutes more. Remove the fish from the air fryer grill to a plate.

7. Assemble the tacos: Spoon some of the coleslaw mix into each tortilla and top each with $1/3$ of a tilapia fillet. Squeeze some lime juice over the top of each taco and serve immediately.

28. Cauliflower and Sole Fritters

Prep time: 5 minutes | Cook time: 24 minutes | Serves 2

½ pound (227 g) sole fillets
½ pound (227 g) mashed cauliflower
½ cup red onion, chopped
1 bell pepper, finely chopped
1 egg, beaten
2 garlic cloves, minced
2 tablespoons fresh parsley, chopped
1 tablespoon olive oil
1 tablespoon coconut aminos
½ teaspoon scotch bonnet pepper, minced
½ teaspoon paprika
Salt and white pepper, to taste
Cooking spray

1.   Spray the air fry basket with cooking spray. Place the sole fillets in the basket.
2.   Place the basket on the air fry position.
3.   Select Air Fry, set temperature to 395ºF (202ºC), and set time to 10 minutes. Flip the fillets halfway through.
4.   When cooking is complete, transfer the fish fillets to a large bowl. Mash the fillets into flakes. Add the remaining ingredients and stir to combine.
5.   Make the fritters: Scoop out 2 tablespoons of the fish mixture and shape into a patty about ½ inch thick with your hands. Repeat with the remaining fish mixture. Place the patties in the air fry basket.
6.   Place the basket on the bake position.
7.   Select Bake, set temperature to 380ºF (193ºC), and set time to 14 minutes. Flip the patties halfway through.
8.   When cooking is complete, they should be golden brown and cooked through. Remove the basket from the air fryer grill and cool for 5 minutes before serving.

29. Crispy Salmon Spring Rolls

Prep time: 20 minutes | Cook time: 18 minutes | Serves 4

½ pound (227 g) salmon fillet
1 teaspoon toasted sesame oil
1 onion, sliced
1 carrot, shredded
1 yellow bell pepper, thinly sliced
$^1/_3$ cup chopped fresh flat-leaf parsley
¼ cup chopped fresh basil
8 rice paper wrappers

1.   Arrange the salmon in the air fry basket. Drizzle the sesame oil all over the salmon and scatter the onion on top.
2.   Place the basket on the air fry position.
3.   Select Air Fry, set temperature to 370ºF (188ºC), and set time to 10 minutes.
4.   Meanwhile, fill a small shallow bowl with warm water. One by one, dip the rice paper wrappers into the water for a few seconds or just until moistened, then put them on a work surface.
5.   When cooking is complete, the fish should flake apart with a fork. Remove from the air fryer grill to a plate.
6.   Make the spring rolls: Place ⅛ of the salmon and onion mixture, bell pepper, carrot, basil, and parsley into the center of the rice wrapper and fold the sides over the filling. Roll up the wrapper carefully and tightly like you would a burrito. Repeat with the remaining wrappers and filling.
7.   Transfer the rolls to the air fry basket.
8.   Place the basket on the bake position.
9.   Select Bake, set temperature to 380ºF (193ºC), and set time to 8 minutes.
10.   When cooking is complete, the rolls should be crispy and lightly browned. Remove from the air fryer grill and cut each roll in half and serve warm.

30. Spiced Red Snapper Fillet

Prep time: 13 minutes | Cook time: 10 minutes | Serves 4

1 teaspoon olive oil
1½ teaspoons black pepper
¼ teaspoon garlic powder
¼ teaspoon thyme
⅛ teaspoon cayenne pepper
4 (4-ounce / 113-g) red snapper fillets, skin on
4 thin slices lemon
Nonstick cooking spray

1.   Spritz the air fry basket with nonstick cooking spray.
2.   In a small bowl, stir together the olive oil, black pepper, thyme, garlic powder, and cayenne

pepper. Rub the mixture all over the fillets until completely coated.

3.   Lay the fillets, skin-side down, in the air fry basket and top each fillet with a slice of lemon.

4.   Place the basket on the bake position.

5.   Select Bake, set temperature to 390ºF (199ºC), and set time to 10 minutes. Flip the fillets halfway through.

6.   When cooking is complete, the fish should be cooked through. Let the fish cool for 5 minutes and serve.

31. .Fruity Sweet-Sour Snapper Fillet

Prep time: 15 minutes | Cook time: 12 minutes | Serves 4

4 (4-ounce / 113-g) red snapper fillets
2 teaspoons olive oil
3 plums, halved and pitted
3 nectarines, halved and pitted
1 cup red grapes
1 tablespoon freshly squeezed lemon juice
1 tablespoon honey
½ teaspoon dried thyme

1.   Arrange the red snapper fillets in the air fry basket and drizzle the olive oil over the top.

2.   Place the basket on the air fry position.

3.   Select Air Fry, set temperature to 390ºF (199ºC), and set time to 12 minutes.

4.   After 4 minutes, remove the basket from the air fryer grill. Top the fillets with the plums and nectarines. Scatter the red grapes all over the fillets. Drizzle with the honey and lemon juice and sprinkle the thyme on top. Return the basket to the air fryer grill and continue cooking for 8 minutes, or until the fish is flaky.

5.   When cooking is complete, remove from the air fryer grill and serve warm.

32. Gold Salmon Patties

Prep time: 5 minutes | Cook time: 11 minutes | Makes 6 patties

1 (14.75-ounce / 418-g) can Alaskan pink salmon, drained and bones removed
½ cup bread crumbs
1 egg, whisked
2 scallions, diced
1 teaspoon garlic powder
Salt and pepper, to taste
Cooking spray

1.   Stir together the salmon, bread crumbs, whisked egg, garlic powder, scallions, salt, and pepper in a large bowl until well incorporated.

2.   Divide the salmon mixture into six equal portions and form each into a patty with your hands.

3.   Arrange the salmon patties in the air fry basket and spritz them with cooking spray.

4.   Place the basket on the air fry position.

5.   Air Fry, set temperature to 400ºF (205ºC), and set time to 10 minutes. Flip the patties once halfway through.

6.   When cooking is complete, the patties should be golden brown and cooked through. Remove the patties from the air fryer grill and serve on a plate.

33. Toasted Salmon with Asparagus

Prep time: 10 minutes | Cook time: 15 minutes | Serves 4

4 (6-ounce / 170 g) salmon fillets, patted dry
1 teaspoon kosher salt, divided
1 tablespoon honey
2 tablespoons unsalted butter, melted
2 teaspoons Dijon mustard
2 pounds (907 g) asparagus, trimmed
Lemon wedges, for serving

1.   Season both sides of the salmon fillets with ½ teaspoon of kosher salt.

2.   Whisk together the honey, 1 tablespoon of butter, and mustard in a small bowl. Set aside.

3.   Arrange the asparagus on a sheet pan. Drizzle the remaining 1 tablespoon of butter all over and season with the remaining ½ teaspoon of salt, tossing to coat. Move the asparagus to the outside of the sheet pan.

4.   Put the salmon fillets on the sheet pan, skin-side down. Brush the fillets generously with the honey mixture.

5.   Place the pan on the toast position.

6.   Select Toast, set temperature to 375ºF (190ºC), and set time to 15 minutes. Toss the asparagus once halfway through the cooking time.

7.   When done, transfer the salmon fillets and asparagus to a plate. Serve warm with a squeeze of lemon juice.

34. Sheet Pan Shrimp Fajitas

Who doesn't love shrimp fajitas? Try out this quick recipe today.

Prep Time and Cooking Time: 20 minutes | Serves: 2

Ingredients to Use:

8 oz. shrimp, deveined and peeled

1 minced garlic clove

2 tbsp. lime juice

1 tbsp. olive oil

Chili pepper & cayenne pepper

Sour cream

2 avocados, sliced

Cilantro, chopped

4 tortillas

Salt and pepper

Step-by-Step Directions to cook it:

1. *Mix all the spices and seasonings and add it to the shrimps.*
2. *Preheat the PowerXL Air Fryer Grill at 177ᵒC or 350ᵒF.*
3. *Bake the shrimps in the pan with chili peppers*
4. *Serve in tortillas*

Nutritional value per serving:

Calories: 408kcal, Carbs: 76g, Protein: 42g, Fat: 6g.

35. Cod Fillets

Prep time: 15 minutes | Cook time: 12 minutes | Serves 4

4 cod fillets

1 teaspoon cayenne pepper

¼ teaspoon fine sea salt

¼ teaspoon ground black pepper, or more to taste

½ cup fresh Italian parsley, coarsely chopped

½ cup non-dairy milk

4 garlic cloves, minced

1 Italian pepper, chopped

1 teaspoon dried basil

½ teaspoon dried oregano

Cooking spray

1. Lightly spritz a baking dish with cooking spray.
2. Season the fillets with cayenne pepper, salt, and black pepper.

3. Pulse the remaining ingredients in a food processor, then transfer the mixture to a shallow bowl. Coat the fillets with the mixture.
4. Place the baking dish into the air fryer grill.
5. Select Air Fry, set temperature to 375ºF (190ºC), and set time to 12 minutes.
6. When cooking is complete, the fish will be flaky. Remove from the air fryer grill and serve on a plate.

36. Baked Cajun Cod

Prep time: 5 minutes | Cook time: 12 minutes | Makes 2 cod fillets

1 tablespoon Cajun seasoning

1 teaspoon salt

½ teaspoon lemon pepper

½ teaspoon freshly ground black pepper

2 (8-ounce / 227-g) cod fillets, cut to fit into the air fry basket

Cooking spray

2 tablespoons unsalted butter, melted

1 lemon, cut into 4 wedges

1. Spritz the air fry basket with cooking spray.
2. Thoroughly combine the Cajun seasoning, lemon pepper, salt, and black pepper in a small bowl. Rub this mixture all over the cod fillets until completely coated.
3. Put the fillets in the air fry basket and brush the melted butter over both sides of each fillet.
4. Place the basket on the bake position.
5. Select Bake, set temperature to 360ºF (182ºC), and set time to 12 minutes. Flip the fillets halfway through the cooking time.
6. When cooking is complete, the fish should flake apart with a fork. Remove the fillets from the air fryer grill and serve with fresh lemon wedges.

37. Crispy Salmon Patties

Prep time: 10 minutes | Cook time: 13 minutes | Serves 4

1 pound (454 g) salmon, chopped into ½-inch pieces

2 tablespoons coconut flour

2 tablespoons grated Parmesan cheese

1½ tablespoons milk

½ white onion, peeled and finely chopped

½ teaspoon butter, at room temperature

½ teaspoon chipotle powder

½ teaspoon dried parsley flakes

$^1/_3$ teaspoon ground black pepper

$^1/_3$ teaspoon smoked cayenne pepper

1 teaspoon fine sea salt

1. Put all the ingredients for the salmon patties in a bowl and stir to combine well.

2. Scoop out 2 tablespoons of the salmon mixture and shape into a patty with your palm, about ½ inch thick. Repeat until all the mixture is used. Transfer to the refrigerator for about 2 hours until firm.

3. When ready, arrange the salmon patties in the air fry basket.

4. Place the basket on the bake position.

5. Select Bake, set temperature to 395ºF (202ºC), and set time to 13 minutes. Flip the patties halfway through the cooking time.

6. When cooking is complete, the patties should be golden brown. Remove from the air fryer grill and cool for 5 minutes before serving.

38. Tuna Casserole

Prep time: 10 minutes | Cook time: 16 minutes | Serves 4

½ tablespoon sesame oil

$^1/_3$ cup yellow onions, chopped

½ bell pepper, deveined and chopped

2 cups canned tuna, chopped

Cooking spray

5 eggs, beaten

½ chili pepper, deveined and finely minced

1½ tablespoons sour cream

$^1/_3$ teaspoon dried basil

$^1/_3$ teaspoon dried oregano

Fine sea salt and ground black pepper, to taste

1. Heat the sesame oil in a nonstick skillet over medium heat until it shimmers.

2. Add the bell pepper and onions and sauté for 4 minutes, stirring occasionally, or until tender.

3. Add the canned tuna and keep stirring until the tuna is heated through.

4. Meanwhile, coat a baking dish lightly with cooking spray.

5. Transfer the tuna mixture to the baking dish, along with the beaten eggs, sour cream, chili pepper, basil, and oregano. Stir to combine well. Season with sea salt and black pepper.

6. Place the baking dish on the bake position.

7. Select Bake, set temperature to 325ºF (160ºC), and set time to 12 minutes.

8. When cooking is complete, the eggs should be completely set and the top lightly browned. Remove from the air fryer grill and serve on a plate.

39. Garlic-Butter Shrimpwith Potatoes

Prep time: 10 minutes | Cook time: 15 minutes | Serves 4

1 pound (454 g) small red potatoes, halved

2 ears corn, shucked and cut into rounds, 1 to 1½ inches thick

2 tablespoons Old Bay or similar seasoning

½ cup unsalted butter, melted

1 (12- to 13-ounce / 340- to 369-g) package kielbasa or other smoked sausages

3 garlic cloves, minced

1 pound (454 g) medium shrimp, peeled and deveined

1. Place the potatoes and corn in a large bowl.

2. Stir together the butter and Old Bay seasoning in a small bowl. Drizzle half the butter mixture over the corn and potatoes, tossing to coat. Spread out the vegetables on a sheet pan.

3. Place the pan on the toast position.

4. Select Toast, set temperature to 350ºF (180ºC), and set time to 15 minutes.

5. Meanwhile, cut the sausages into 2-inch lengths, then cut each piece in half lengthwise. Put the sausages and shrimp in a medium bowl and set aside.

6. Add the garlic to the bowl of remaining butter mixture and stir well.

7. After 10 minutes, remove the sheet pan and pour the vegetables into the large bowl. Drizzle with the toss and garlic butter until well coated. Arrange the vegetables, sausages, and shrimp on the sheet pan.

8. Return to the air fryer grill and continue cooking. After 5 minutes, check the shrimp for doneness. The shrimp should be pink and opaque. If they are not quite cooked through, roast for an additional 1 minute.

9. When done, remove from the air fryer grill and serve on a plate.

40. Easy Salmon Patties

Prep time: 5 minutes | Cook time: 11 minutes | Makes 6 patties

1 (14.75-ounce / 418-g) can Alaskan pink salmon, drained and bones removed
½ cup bread crumbs
1 egg, whisked
2 scallions, diced
1 teaspoon garlic powder
Salt and pepper, to taste
Cooking spray

1. Stir together the salmon, bread crumbs, whisked egg, scallions, garlic powder, salt, and pepper in a large bowl until well incorporated.
2. Divide the salmon mixture into six equal portions and form each into a patty with your hands.
3. Arrange the salmon patties in the air fry basket and spritz them with cooking spray.
4. Select Air Fry, Super Convection, set temperature to 400ºF (205ºC), and set time to 10 minutes. Select Start/Stop to begin preheating.
5. Once preheated, place the basket on the air fry position. Flip the patties once halfway through.
6. When cooking is complete, the patties should be golden brown and cooked through. Remove the patties from the oven and serve on a plate.

41. Broiled Crab Cakes With Herb Sauce

This crab cake makes for a perfect afternoon snack.
Prep Time and Cooking Time: 25 minutes | Serves: 4
Ingredients to use:
1 lb. crab meat
1 large egg
1 minced garlic clove
1/4 parsley, chopped
1 tsp. seafood seasoning
Salt & pepper
1 shallot
1 tbsp. brown mustard
4 tbsp. mayo
1 tbsp. flour
Step-by-Step Directions to cook it:
1. Mix mayo, eggs, mustard, seasoning, and flour until smooth

2. Stir in the lump of crab meat along with shallots, parsley, garlic.
3. Make 4 balls and place them on the pan
4. Broil in the PowerXL Air Fryer Grill at 121C or 250ºF for 8 minutes.
Nutritional value per serving:
Calories: 240kcal, Carbs: 8g, Protein: 16g, Fat: 16g.

42. .Lemon-Honey Snapper with Fruit

Prep time: 15 minutes | Cook time: 12 minutes | Serves 4

4 (4-ounce / 113-g) red snapper fillets
2 teaspoons olive oil
3 plums, halved and pitted
3 nectarines, halved and pitted
1 cup red grapes
1 tablespoon freshly squeezed lemon juice
1 tablespoon honey
½ teaspoon dried thyme

1. Arrange the red snapper fillets in the air fry basket and drizzle the olive oil over the top.
2. Select Air Fry, Super Convection, set temperature to 390ºF (199ºC), and set time to 12 minutes. Select Start/Stop to begin preheating.
3. Once preheated, place the basket on the air fry position.
4. After 4 minutes, remove the basket from the oven. Top the fillets with the plums and nectarines. Scatter the red grapes all over the fillets. Drizzle with the lemon juice and honey and sprinkle the thyme on top. Return the basket to the oven and continue cooking for 8 minutes, or until the fish is flaky.
5. When cooking is complete, remove from the oven and serve warm.

43. Asian-Inspired Swordfish Steaks

Prep time: 10 minutes | Cook time: 8 minutes | Serves 4

4 (4-ounce / 113-g) swordfish steaks
½ teaspoon toasted sesame oil
1 jalapeño pepper, finely minced
2 garlic cloves, grated
2 tablespoons freshly squeezed lemon juice
1 tablespoon grated fresh ginger
½ teaspoon Chinese five-spice powder
⅛ teaspoon freshly ground black pepper

1. On a clean work surface, place the swordfish steaks and brush both sides of the fish with the sesame oil.
2. Combine the jalapeño, garlic, lemon juice, ginger, five-spice powder, and black pepper in a small bowl and stir to mix well. Rub the mixture all over the fish until completely coated. Allow to sit for 10 minutes.
3. When ready, arrange the swordfish steaks in the air fry basket.
4. Select Air Fry, Super Convection, set temperature to 380ºF (193ºC), and set time to 8 minutes. Select Start/Stop to begin preheating.
5. Once preheated, place the basket on the air fry position. Flip the steaks halfway through.
6. When cooking is complete, remove from the oven and cool for 5 minutes before serving.

44. Baked Sole with Asparagus

Ending the seafood chapter with this fantastic baked Sole recipe.
Prep Time and Cooking Time: 25 minutes | Serves: 4
Ingredients to use:
2 lbs. asparagus
1 tsp. olive oil
3 tbsp. parmesan, grated
Salt and black pepper
2 tbsp. panko breadcrumbs
1 tsp. minced chives
2 tbsp. mayo
2 fillets of sole, 8 oz.
1/4 lemon, cut into wedges
Step-by-Step Directions to cook it:
1. **Preheat the PowerXL Air Fryer Grill at 232ºC or 450ºF.**
2. **Season the asparagus with olive oil and seasoning**
3. **Mix breadcrumbs, cheese, salt, and pepper.**
4. **Mix mayo with chives and brush this on to the fillets**
5. **Press the brushed sides with the cheese mix**
6. **Bake for 15 minutes. Serve with lemon juice.**
Nutritional value per serving:
Calories: 284kcal, Carbs: 18g, Protein: 35g, Fat: 9g.

45. Butter-Wine Baked Salmon

Prep time: 5 minutes | Cook time: 10 minutes | Serves 4
4 tablespoons butter, melted
2 cloves garlic, minced
Sea salt and ground black pepper, to taste
¼ cup dry white wine
1 tablespoon lime juice
1 teaspoon smoked paprika
½ teaspoon onion powder
4 salmon steaks
Cooking spray
1. Place all the ingredients except the salmon and oil in a shallow dish and stir to mix well.
2. Add the salmon steaks, turning to coat well on both sides. Transfer the salmon to the refrigerator to marinate for 30 minutes.
3. When ready, put the salmon steaks in the air fry basket, discarding any excess marinade. Spray the salmon steaks with cooking spray.
4. Select Air Fry, Super Convection, set temperature to 360ºF (182ºC), and set time to 10 minutes. Select Start/Stop to begin preheating.
5. Once preheated, place the basket on the air fry position. Flip the salmon steaks halfway through.
6. When cooking is complete, remove from the oven and divide the salmon steaks among four plates. Serve warm.

46. Broiled Chipotle Tilapia

Try out this amazing seafood chipotle with delicious Tilapia.
Prep Time and Cooking Time: 20 minutes | Serves: 2
Ingredients to use:
1/2 lbs. tilapia fillets
1 tsp. lime juice
Cilantro, chopped
3 tsp. chipotle
1 avocado, peeled and halved
3 tbsp. sour cream
Mayo, 1 tbsp.
Step-by-Step Directions to cook it:
1. *Blend the ingredients except for the fish.*
2. *Brush the fish fillets with the mix.*
3. *Broil the fish at 132ºC or 270ºF in the PowerXL Air Fryer Grill for 10 minutes.*

Nutritional value per serving:
Calories: 385kcal, Carbs: 65g, Protein: 18g, Fat: 7g,

47. Golden Beer-Battered Cod

Prep time: 5 minutes | Cook time: 15 minutes | Serves 4

2 eggs
1 cup malty beer
1 cup all-purpose flour
½ cup cornstarch
1 teaspoon garlic powder
Salt and pepper, to taste
4 (4-ounce / 113-g) cod fillets
Cooking spray

1.   In a shallow bowl, beat together the eggs with the beer. In another shallow bowl, thoroughly combine the flour and cornstarch. Sprinkle with the garlic powder, salt, and pepper.
2.   Dredge each cod fillet in the flour mixture, then in the egg mixture. Dip each piece of fish in the flour mixture a second time.
3.   Spritz the air fry basket with cooking spray. Arrange the cod fillets in the basket in a single layer.
4.   Select Air Fry, Super Convection, set temperature to 400ºF (205ºC), and set time to 15 minutes. Select Start/Stop to begin preheating.
5.   Once preheated, place the basket on the air fry position. Flip the fillets halfway through the cooking time.
6.   When cooking is complete, the cod should reach an internal temperature of 145ºF (63ºC) on a meat thermometer and the outside should be crispy. Let the fish cool for 5 minutes and serve.

48. Garlicky Cod Fillets

Prep time: 10 minutes | Cook time: 12 minutes | Serves 4

1 teaspoon olive oil
4 cod fillets
¼ teaspoon fine sea salt
¼ teaspoon ground black pepper, or more to taste
1 teaspoon cayenne pepper
½ cup fresh Italian parsley, coarsely chopped
½ cup nondairy milk
1 Italian pepper, chopped
4 garlic cloves, minced
1 teaspoon dried basil

½ teaspoon dried oregano

1.   Lightly coat the sides and bottom of a baking dish with the olive oil. Set aside.
2.   In a large bowl, sprinkle the fillets with salt, black pepper, and cayenne pepper.
3.   In a food processor, pulse the remaining ingredients until smoothly puréed.
4.   Add the purée to the bowl of fillets and toss to coat, then transfer to the prepared baking dish.
5.   Select Bake, Super Convection, set temperature to 380ºF (193ºC), and set time to 12 minutes. Select Start/Stop to begin preheating.
6.   Once preheated, place the baking dish on the bake position.
7.   When cooking is complete, the fish should flake when pressed lightly with a fork. Remove from the oven and serve warm.

49. Dijon Salmon with Green Beans

Check out one of the best salmon dish recipes.
Prep Time and Cooking Time: 30 minutes | Serves: 2-3

Ingredients to use

1 tbsp. dijon mustard
3/4 lbs. salmon fillets
1 tbsp. soy sauce
2 garlic cloves
1/2 small red bell pepper, sliced
Salt and pepper
2 tbsp. olive oil
6 oz. green beans, trimmed
1 small leek, sliced

Step-by-Step Directions to cook it:

1.   *Preheat the PowerXL Air Fryer Grill to 204ºC or 400ºF.*
2.   *Mix soy sauce, olive oil, garlic, and mustard.*
3.   *Mix the remaining ingredients with olive oil.*
4.   *Place the salmon fillets, brushed with the oil mix, on the pan with the veggies around*
5.   *Bake for 15 minutes.*

Nutritional value per serving:
Calories: 295kcal, Carbs: 5g, Protein: 23g, Fat: 20g.

50. Lemony Gold Sole

Prep time: 5 minutes | Cook time: 10 minutes | Serves 4

5 teaspoons low-sodium yellow mustard
1 tablespoon freshly squeezed lemon juice
4 (3.5-ounce / 99-g) sole fillets
2 teaspoons olive oil
½ teaspoon dried marjoram
½ teaspoon dried thyme
⅛ teaspoon freshly ground black pepper
1 slice low-sodium whole-wheat bread, crumbled

1.   Whisk together the mustard and lemon juice in a small bowl until thoroughly mixed and smooth. Spread the mixture evenly over the sole fillets, then transfer the fillets to the air fry basket.
2.   In a separate bowl, combine the olive oil, black pepper, thyme, marjoram, and bread crumbs and stir to mix well. Gently but firmly press the mixture onto the top of fillets, coating them completely.
3.   Place the basket on the bake position.
4.   Select Bake, set temperature to 320ºF (160ºC), and set time to 10 minutes.
5.   When cooking is complete, the fish should reach an internal temperature of 145ºF (63ºC) on a meat thermometer. Remove the basket from the air fryer grill and serve on a plate.

51. .Spicy Shrimp

Prep time: 5 minutes | Cook time: 10 minutes | Serves 4

1 pound (454 g) tiger shrimp
2 tablespoons olive oil
½ tablespoon old bay seasoning
¼ tablespoon smoked paprika
¼ teaspoon cayenne pepper
A pinch of sea salt

1.   Toss all the ingredients in a large bowl until the shrimp are evenly coated.
2.   Arrange the shrimp in the air fry basket.
3.   Place the basket on the air fry position.
4.   Select Air Fry, set temperature to 380ºF (193ºC), and set time to 10 minutes.
5.   When cooking is complete, the shrimp should be pink and cooked through. Remove from the air fryer grill and serve hot.

52. Pecan-Crusted Catfish

Prep time: 5 minutes | Cook time: 12 minutes | Serves 4

½ cup pecan meal
1 teaspoon fine sea salt
¼ teaspoon ground black pepper
4 (4-ounce / 113-g) catfish fillets
Avocado oil spray
For Garnish (Optional):
Fresh oregano
Pecan halves

1.   Spray the air fry basket with avocado oil spray.
2.   Combine the sea salt, black pepper and pecan meal in a large bowl. Dredge each catfish fillet in the meal mixture, turning until well coated. Spritz the fillets with avocado oil spray, then transfer to the air fry basket.
3.   Place the basket on the air fry position.
4.   Select Air Fry, set temperature to 375ºF (190ºC), and set time to 12 minutes. Flip the fillets halfway through the cooking time.
5.   When cooking is complete, the fish should be cooked through and no longer translucent. Remove from the air fryer grill and sprinkle the oregano sprigs and pecan halves on top for garnish, if desired. Serve immediately.

53. Tilapia Meunière

Prep time: 10 minutes | Cook time: 20 minutes | Serves 4

10 ounces (283 g) Yukon Gold potatoes, sliced ¼-inch thick
5 tablespoons unsalted butter, melted, divided
1 teaspoon kosher salt, divided
4 (8-ounce / 227-g) tilapia fillets
½ pound (227 g) green beans, trimmed
Juice of 1 lemon
2 tablespoons chopped fresh parsley, for garnish

1.   In a large bowl, drizzle the potatoes with ¼ teaspoon of kosher salt and 2 tablespoons of melted butter. Transfer the potatoes to the sheet pan.
2.   Place the pan on the toast position.
3.   Select Toast, set temperature to 375ºF (190ºC), and set time to 20 minutes.
4.   Meanwhile, season both sides of the fillets with ½ teaspoon of kosher salt. Put the green beans in the medium bowl and sprinkle with the remaining

¼ teaspoon of kosher salt and 1 tablespoon of butter, tossing to coat.

5.   After 10 minutes, remove the pan and push the potatoes to one side. Put the fillets in the middle of the pan and add the green beans on the other side. Drizzle the remaining 2 tablespoons of butter over the fillets. Return the pan to the air fryer grill and continue cooking, or until the fish flakes easily with a fork and the green beans are crisp-tender.

6.   When cooked, remove the pan from the air fryer grill. Drizzle the lemon juice over the fillets and sprinkle the parsley on top for garnish. Serve hot.

54. Garlicky Parmesan-Crusted Hake Fillet

Prep time: 5 minutes | Cook time: 10 minutes | Serves 3
Fish:
6 tablespoons mayonnaise
1 tablespoon fresh lime juice
1 teaspoon Dijon mustard
1 cup grated Parmesan cheese
Salt, to taste
¼ teaspoon ground black pepper, or more to taste
3 hake fillets, patted dry
Nonstick cooking spray
Garlic Sauce:
¼ cup plain Greek yogurt
2 tablespoons olive oil
2 cloves garlic, minced
½ teaspoon minced tarragon leaves

1.   Mix the mayo, lime juice, and mustard in a shallow bowl and whisk to combine. In another shallow bowl, stir together the grated Parmesan cheese, salt, and pepper.
2.   Dredge each fillet in the mayo mixture, then roll them in the cheese mixture until they are evenly coated on both sides.
3.   Spray the air fry basket with nonstick cooking spray. Place the fillets in the basket.
4.   Place the basket on the air fry position.
5.   Select Air Fry, set temperature to 395ºF (202ºC), and set time to 10 minutes. Flip the fillets halfway through the cooking time.
6.   Meanwhile, in a small bowl, whisk all the ingredients for the sauce until well incorporated.

7.   When cooking is complete, the fish should flake apart with a fork. Remove the fillets from the air fryer grill and serve warm alongside the sauce.

55. Fish and Chips

Here's some plain old fish and chips, the classic snack.
Prep Time and Cooking Time: 1 hour | Serves: 4
Ingredients to use:
4 pieces of cod, 6 oz. each
8 thyme sprigs
1-3/4 lb. potato, cubed
1 lemon, cut in half
2 tbsp. capers
Salt & pepper
1 garlic clove
4 tbsp. olive oil
Step-by-Step Directions to cook it:
1.   Preheat the PowerXL Air Fryer Grill to 232 <u>0</u>C or 450 <u>0</u>F.
2.   Bake the potatoes, olive oil, salt, pepper, and 4 thyme sprigs for 30 minutes.
3.   Brush the cod with lemon and put the remaining ingredients on top of the cod
4.   Drizzle some olive oil and bake for another 12 minutes.
Nutritional value per serving:
Calories: 378kcal, Carbs: 33g, Protein: 34g, Fat: 12g.

56. Air-Fryer Scallops with Lemon-Herb Sauce

Prep/Cook Time: 20 mins, Servings: 2
Ingredients
•   8 large (1-oz.) sea scallops, cleaned and patted very dry
•   ¼ teaspoon ground pepper
•   ⅛ teaspoon salt
•   cooking spray
•   ¼ cup extra-virgin olive oil
•   2 tablespoons very finely chopped flat-leaf parsley
•   2 teaspoons capers, very finely chopped
•   1 teaspoon finely grated lemon zest
•   ½ teaspoon finely chopped garlic
•   lemon wedges, optional
Instructions

- Sprinkle scallops with pepper and salt. Coat the basket of an air fryer with cooking spray. Place scallops in the basket and coat them with cooking spray. Place the basket in the fryer. Cook the scallops at 400°F until they reach an internal temperature of 120°F, about 6 minutes.
- Combine oil, parsley, capers, lemon zest and garlic in a small bowl. Drizzle over the scallops. Serve with lemon wedges, if desired.

Nutrition Info
348 calories; total fat 30g; saturated fat 4g; cholesterol 27mg; sodium 660mg; potassium 260mg; carbohydrates 5g;

57. Air Fryer Mahi Mahi with Brown Butter

Prep/Cook Time: 20 mins, Servings: 4

Ingredients
- 4 (6 ounce) mahi mahi fillets
- salt and ground black pepper to taste
- cooking spray
- ⅔ cup butter

Instructions
- Preheat an air fryer to 350 degrees F (175 degrees C).
- Season mahi mahi fillets with salt and pepper and spray with cooking spray on both sides. Place fillets in the air fryer basket, making sure to leave space in between.
- Cook until fish flakes easily with a fork and has a golden hue, about 12 minutes.
- While fish is cooking, melt butter in a small saucepan over medium-low heat. Bring butter to a simmer and cook until butter turns frothy and a rich brown color, 3 to 5 minutes. Remove from heat.
- Transfer fish fillets to a plate and drizzle with brown butter.

Nutrition Info
416 calories; protein 31.8g; carbohydratesg; fat 31.9g; cholesterol 205.4mg; sodium 406.3mg

58. Mustard Crusted Salmon

Here's another variation of the classic salmon fillet.
Prep Time And Cooking Time: 25 minutes | Serves: 4
Ingredients to use:
1 tsp. Dijon mustard

6 oz. salmon filets
1 tsp. chives, chopped
1 tbsp. lemon juice
2 tbsp. sour cream
Salt and pepper
1 tbsp. breadcrumbs (panko)

Step-by-Step Directions to cook it:
1. Preheat the PowerXL Air Fryer Grill at 190°C or 375°F with broil mode.
2. Season the fillets with salt, pepper, and dijon mustard.
3. Sprinkle breadcrumbs on top
4. Bake for 8-9 minutes
5. Serve with sour cream and lemon juice

Nutritional value per serving:
Calories: 350kcal, Carbs: 7g, Protein: 36g, Fat: 19g.

59. Cheesy Shrimp

Prep time: 15 minutes | Cook time: 8 minutes | Serves 2

1 pound (454 g) shrimp, deveined
1½ tablespoons olive oil
1½ tablespoons balsamic vinegar
1 tablespoon coconut aminos
½ tablespoon fresh parsley, roughly chopped
Sea salt flakes, to taste
1 teaspoon Dijon mustard
½ teaspoon smoked cayenne pepper
½ teaspoon garlic powder
Salt and ground black peppercorns, to taste
1 cup shredded goat cheese

1. Except for the cheese, stir together all the ingredients in a large bowl until the shrimp are evenly coated.
2. Place the shrimp in the air fry basket.
3. Place the basket on the toast position.
4. Select Toast, set temperature to 385ºF (196ºC), and set time to 8 minutes.
5. When cooking is complete, the shrimp should be pink and cooked through. Remove from the air fryer grill and serve with the shredded goat cheese sprinkled on top.

60. Hoisin Tuna with Jasmine Rice

Prep time: 15 minutes | Cook time: 5 minutes | Serves 4

½ cup hoisin sauce

2 tablespoons rice wine vinegar

2 teaspoons sesame oil

2 teaspoons dried lemongrass

1 teaspoon garlic powder

¼ teaspoon red pepper flakes

½ small onion, quartered and thinly sliced

8 ounces (227 g) fresh tuna, cut into 1-inch cubes

Cooking spray

3 cups cooked jasmine rice

1.   In a small bowl, whisk together the vinegar, hoisin sauce, sesame oil, garlic powder, lemongrass, and red pepper flakes.

2.   Add the sliced onion and tuna cubes and gently toss until the fish is evenly coated.

3.   Arrange the coated tuna cubes in the air fry basket in a single layer.

4.   Place the basket on the air fry position.

5.   Select Air Fry, set temperature to 390ºF (199ºC), and set time to 5 minutes. Flip the fish halfway through the cooking time.

6.   When cooking is complete, the fish should begin to flake. Continue cooking for 1 minute, if necessary. Remove from the air fryer grill and serve over hot jasmine rice.

61. .Golden Fish Sticks

Prep time: 10 minutes | Cook time: 6 minutes | Serves 8

8 ounces (227 g) fish fillets (pollock or cod), cut into ½ × 3 inches strips

Salt, to taste (optional)

½ cup plain bread crumbs

Cooking spray

1.   Season the fish strips with salt to taste, if desired.

2.   Place the bread crumbs on a plate, then roll the fish in the bread crumbs until well coated. Spray all sides of the fish with cooking spray. Transfer to the air fry basket in a single layer.

3.   Place the basket on the air fry position.

4.   Select Air Fry, set temperature to 400ºF (205ºC), and set time to 6 minutes.

5.   When cooked, the fish sticks should be golden brown and crispy. Remove from the air fryer grill to a plate and serve hot.

62. Panko-Crusted Fish Sticks

Prep time: 10 minutes | Cook time: 8 minutes | Makes 8 fish sticks

8 ounces (227 g) fish fillets (pollock or cod), cut into ½×3-inch strips

Salt, to taste (optional)

½ cup plain bread crumbs

Cooking spray

1.   Season the fish strips with salt to taste, if desired.

2.   Place the bread crumbs on a plate. Roll the fish strips in the bread crumbs to coat. Spritz the fish strips with cooking spray.

3.   Arrange the fish strips in the air fry basket in a single layer.

4.   Place the basket on the air fry position.

5.   Air Fry, set temperature to 390ºF (199ºC), and set time to 8 minutes.

6.   When cooking is complete, they should be golden brown. Remove from the air fryer grill and cool for 5 minutes before serving.

63. Southern Salmon Bowl

Prep time: 115 minutes | Cook time: 12 minutes | Serves 4

12 ounces (340 g) salmon fillets, cut into 1½-inch cubes

1 red onion, chopped

1 jalapeño pepper, minced

1 red bell pepper, chopped

¼ cup low-sodium salsa

2 teaspoons peanut oil or safflower oil

2 tablespoons low-sodium tomato juice

1 teaspoon chili powder

1.   Mix together the salmon cubes, red onion, red bell pepper, jalapeño, peanut oil, tomato juice, salsa, chili powder in a medium metal bowl and stir until well incorporated.

2.   Place the metal bowl on the bake position.

3.   Select Bake, set temperature to 370ºF (188ºC), and set time to 12 minutes. Stir the ingredients once halfway through the cooking time.

4.   When cooking is complete, the salmon should be cooked through and the veggies should be fork-tender. Serve warm.

64. Panko-Crusted Calamari with Lemon

Prep time: 5 minutes | Cook time: 12 minutes | Serves 4

2 large eggs

2 garlic cloves, minced

½ cup cornstarch

1 cup bread crumbs

1 pound (454 g) calamari rings

Cooking spray

1 lemon, sliced

1.   In a small bowl, whisk the eggs with minced garlic. Place the bread crumbs and cornstarch into separate shallow dishes.

2.   Dredge the calamari rings in the cornstarch, then dip in the egg mixture, shaking off any excess, finally roll them in the bread crumbs to coat well. Let the calamari rings sit for 10 minutes in the refrigerator.

3.   Spritz the air fry basket with cooking spray. Transfer the calamari rings to the basket.

4.   Place the basket on the air fry position.

5.   Select Air Fry, set temperature to 390ºF (199ºC), and set time to 12 minutes. Stir the calamari rings once halfway through the cooking time.

6.   When cooking is complete, remove the basket from the air fryer grill. Serve the calamari rings with the lemon slices sprinkled on top.

65. Lemony Shrimp with Parsley

Prep time: 10 minutes | Cook time: 5 minutes | Serves 4

18 shrimp, shelled and deveined

2 garlic cloves, peeled and minced

2 tablespoons extra-virgin olive oil

2 tablespoons freshly squeezed lemon juice

½ cup fresh parsley, coarsely chopped

1 teaspoon onion powder

1 teaspoon lemon-pepper seasoning

½ teaspoon hot paprika

½ teaspoon salt

¼ teaspoon cumin powder

1.   Toss all the ingredients in a mixing bowl until the shrimp are well coated.

2.   Cover and allow to marinate in the refrigerator for 30 minutes.

3.   When ready, transfer the shrimp to the air fry basket.

4.   Place the basket on the air fry position.

5.   Select Air Fry, set temperature to 400ºF (205ºC), and set time to 5 minutes.

6.   When cooking is complete, the shrimp should be pink on the outside and opaque in the center. Remove from the air fryer grill and serve warm.

66. Fast Bacon-Wrapped Scallops

Prep time: 5 minutes | Cook time: 10 minutes | Serves 4

8 slices bacon, cut in half

16 sea scallops, patted dry

Cooking spray

Salt and freshly ground black pepper, to taste

16 toothpicks, soaked in water for at least 30 minutes

1.   On a clean work surface, wrap half of a slice of bacon around each scallop and secure with a toothpick.

2.   Lay the bacon-wrapped scallops in the air fry basket in a single layer.

3.   Spritz the scallops with cooking spray and sprinkle the salt and pepper to season.

4.   Place the basket on the air fry position.

5.   Select Air Fry, set temperature to 370ºF (188ºC), and set time to 10 minutes. Flip the scallops halfway through the cooking time.

6.   When cooking is complete, the bacon should be cooked through and the scallops should be firm. Remove the scallops from the air fryer grill to a plate Serve warm.

67. Panko-Crusted Catfish Nuggets

Prep time: 10 minutes | Cook time: 7 to 8 minutes | Serves 4

2 medium catfish fillets, cut into chunks (approximately 1 × 2 inch)

Salt and pepper, to taste

2 eggs

2 tablespoons skim milk

½ cup cornstarch

1 cup panko bread crumbs

Cooking spray

1.   In a medium bowl, season the fish chunks with salt and pepper to taste.

2.   In a small bowl, beat together the eggs with milk until well combined.

3. Place the cornstarch and bread crumbs into separate shallow dishes.

4. Dredge the fish chunks one at a time in the cornstarch, coating well on both sides, then dip in the egg mixture, shaking off any excess, finally press well into the bread crumbs. Spritz the fish chunks with cooking spray.

5. Arrange the fish chunks in the air fry basket in a single layer.

6. Place the basket on the air fry position.

7. Select Air Fry, set temperature to 390ºF (199ºC), and set time to 8 minutes. Flip the fish chunks halfway through the cooking time.

8. When cooking is complete, they should be no longer translucent in the center and golden brown. Remove the fish chunks from the air fryer grill to a plate. Serve warm.

68. Lemony Tilapia Fillet

Prep time: 10 minutes | Cook time: 12 minutes | Serves 4

1 tablespoon olive oil
1 tablespoon lemon juice
1 teaspoon minced garlic
½ teaspoon chili powder
4 tilapia fillets

1. Line a baking pan with parchment paper.

2. In a shallow bowl, stir together the lemon juice, olive oil, chili powder, and garlic to make a marinade. Put the tilapia fillets in the bowl, turning to coat evenly.

3. Place the fillets in the baking pan in a single layer.

4. Slide the pan into the air fryer grill.

5. Select Air Fry, set temperature to 375ºF (190ºC), and set time to 12 minutes.

6. When cooked, the fish will flake apart with a fork. Remove from the air fryer grill to a plate and serve hot.

69. .Coconut Spicy Fish

Prep time: 10 minutes | Cook time: 22 minutes | Serves 4

2 tablespoons sunflower oil, divided
1 pound (454 g) fish, chopped
1 ripe tomato, pureéd
2 red chilies, chopped
1 shallot, minced
1 garlic clove, minced
1 cup coconut milk
1 tablespoon coriander powder
1 teaspoon red curry paste
½ teaspoon fenugreek seeds
Salt and white pepper, to taste

1. Coat the air fry basket with 1 tablespoon of sunflower oil. Place the fish in the air fry basket.

2. Place the basket on the air fry position.

3. Select Air Fry, set temperature to 380ºF (193ºC), and set time to 10 minutes. Flip the fish halfway through the cooking time.

4. When cooking is complete, transfer the cooked fish to a baking pan greased with the remaining 1 tablespoon of sunflower oil. Stir in the remaining ingredients.

5. Place the pan on the air fry position.

6. Select Air Fry, set temperature to 350ºF (180ºC), and set time to 12 minutes.

7. When cooking is complete, they should be heated through. Cool for 5 to 8 minutes before serving.

70. Lemony Parsley Shrimp

Prep time: 10 minutes | Cook time: 8 minutes | Serves 4

1 pound (454 g) shrimp, deveined
4 tablespoons olive oil
1½ tablespoons lemon juice
1½ tablespoons fresh parsley, roughly chopped
2 cloves garlic, finely minced
1 teaspoon crushed red pepper flakes, or more to taste
Garlic pepper, to taste
Sea salt flakes, to taste

1. Toss all the ingredients in a large bowl until the shrimp are coated on all sides.

2. Arrange the shrimp in the air fry basket.

3. Place the basket on the air fry position.

4. Select Air Fry, set temperature to 385ºF (196ºC), and set time to 8 minutes.

5. When cooking is complete, the shrimp should be pink and cooked through. Remove from the air fryer grill and serve warm.

71. Toasted Nicoise Salad

Prep time: 10 minutes | Cook time: 15 minutes | Serves 4

10 ounces (283 g) small red potatoes, quartered

8 tablespoons extra-virgin olive oil, divided

1 teaspoon kosher salt, divided

½ pound (227 g) green beans, trimmed

1 pint cherry tomatoes

1 teaspoon Dijon mustard

3 tablespoons red wine vinegar

Freshly ground black pepper, to taste

1 (9-ounce / 255-g) bag spring greens, washed and dried if needed

2 (5-ounce / 142-g) cans oil-packed tuna, drained

2 hard-cooked eggs, peeled and quartered

$^1/_3$ cup kalamata olives, pitted

1.   In a large bowl, drizzle the potatoes with 1 tablespoon of olive oil and season with ¼ teaspoon of kosher salt. Transfer to a sheet pan.

2.   Place the pan on the toast position.

3.   Select Toast, set temperature to 375ºF (190ºC), and set time to 15 minutes.

4.   Meanwhile, in a mixing bowl, toss the green beans and cherry tomatoes with 1 tablespoon of olive oil and ¼ teaspoon of kosher salt until evenly coated.

5.   After 10 minutes, remove the pan and fold in the green beans and cherry tomatoes. Return the pan to the air fryer grill and continue cooking.

6.   Meanwhile, make the vinaigrette by whisking together the remaining 6 tablespoons of olive oil, mustard, vinegar, the remaining ½ teaspoon of kosher salt, and black pepper in a small bowl. Set aside.

7.   When done, remove the pan from the air fryer grill. Allow the vegetables to cool for 5 minutes.

8.   Spread out the spring greens on a plate and spoon the tuna into the center of the greens. Arrange the potatoes, green beans, cheery tomatoes, and eggs around the tuna. Serve drizzled with the vinaigrette and scattered with the olives.

72. Shrimp Saladwith Caesar Dressing

Prep time: 10 minutes | Cook time: 15 minutes | Serves 4

½ baguette, cut into 1-inch cubes (about 2½ cups)

4 tablespoons extra-virgin olive oil, divided

¼ teaspoon granulated garlic

¼ teaspoon kosher salt

¾ cup Caesar dressing , divided

2 romaine lettuce hearts, cut in half lengthwise and ends trimmed

1 pound (454 g) medium shrimp, peeled and deveined

2 ounces (57 g) Parmesan cheese, coarsely grated

1.   Make the croutons: Put the bread cubes in a medium bowl and drizzle 3 tablespoons of olive oil over top. Season with salt and granulated garlic and toss to coat. Transfer to the air fry basket in a single layer.

2.   Place the basket on the air fry position.

3.   Select Air Fry, set temperature to 400ºF (205ºC), and set time to 4 minutes. Toss the croutons halfway through the cooking time.

4.   When done, remove the air fry basket from the air fryer grill and set aside.

5.   Brush 2 tablespoons of Caesar dressing on the cut side of the lettuce . Set aside.

6.   Toss the shrimp with the ¼ cup of Caesar dressing in a large bowl until well coated. Set aside.

7.   Coat the sheet pan with the remaining 1 tablespoon of olive oil. Arrange the romaine halves on the coated pan, cut side down. Brush the tops with the remaining 2 tablespoons of Caesar dressing.

8.   Place the pan on the toast position.

9.   Select Toast, set temperature to 375ºF (190ºC), and set time to 10 minutes.

10.   After 5 minutes, remove the pan from the air fryer grill and flip the romaine halves. Spoon the shrimp around the lettuce. Return the pan to the air fryer grill and continue cooking.

11.   When done, remove the sheet pan from the air fryer grill. If they are not quite cooked through, roast for another 1 minute.

12.   On each of four plates, put a romaine half. Divide the shrimp among the plates and top with croutons and grated Parmesan cheese. Serve immediately.

73. Tuna Patties with Cheese Sauced

Prep time: 5 minutes | Cook time: 17 to 18 minutes | Serves 4

Tuna Patties:

1 pound (454 g) canned tuna, drained

1 egg, whisked

2 tablespoons shallots, minced

1 garlic clove, minced

1 cup grated Romano cheese

Sea salt and ground black pepper, to taste

1 tablespoon sesame oil

Cheese Sauce:

1 tablespoon butter

1 cup beer

2 tablespoons grated Colby cheese

1. Mix together the canned tuna, whisked egg, cheese, shallots, salt, and pepper in a large bowl and stir to incorporate.

2. Divide the tuna mixture into four equal portions and form each portion into a patty with your hands. Refrigerate the patties for 2 hours.

3. When ready, brush both sides of each patty with sesame oil, then place in the air fry basket.

4. Place the basket on the bake position.

5. Select Bake, set temperature to 360ºF (182ºC), and set time to 14 minutes. Flip the patties halfway through the cooking time.

6. Meanwhile, melt the butter in a saucepan over medium heat.

7. Pour in the beer and whisk constantly, or until it begins to bubble. Add the grated Colby cheese and mix well. Continue cooking for 3 to 4 minutes, or until the cheese melts. Remove from the heat.

8. When cooking is complete, the patties should be lightly browned and cooked through. Remove the patties from the air fryer grill to a plate. Drizzle them with the cheese sauce and serve immediately.

74. .Cheesy Cajun Catfish Cakes

Prep time: 5 minutes | Cook time: 15 minutes | Serves 4

2 catfish fillets

3 ounces (85 g) butter

1 cup shredded Parmesan cheese

1 cup shredded Swiss cheese

½ cup buttermilk

1 teaspoon baking powder

1 teaspoon baking soda

1 teaspoon Cajun seasoning

1. Bring a pot of salted water to a boil. Add the catfish fillets to the boiling water and let them boil for 5 minutes until they become opaque.

2. Remove the fillets from the pot to a mixing bowl and flake them into small pieces with a fork.

3. Add the remaining ingredients to the bowl of fish and stir until well incorporated.

4. Divide the fish mixture into 12 equal portions and shape each portion into a patty. Place the patties in the air fry basket.

5. Place the basket on the air fry position.

6. Select Air Fry, set temperature to 380ºF (193ºC), and set time to 15 minutes. Flip the patties halfway through the cooking time.

7. When cooking is complete, the patties should be golden brown and cooked through. Remove from the air fryer grill. Let the patties sit for 5 minutes and serve.

75. Garlicky Orange Shrimp

Prep time: 40 minutes | Cook time: 12 minutes | Serves 4

$^1/_3$ cup orange juice

3 teaspoons minced garlic

1 teaspoon Old Bay seasoning

¼ to ½ teaspoon cayenne pepper

1 pound (454 g) medium shrimp, thawed, deveined, peeled, with tails off, and patted dry

Cooking spray

1. Stir together the orange juice, garlic, Old Bay seasoning, and cayenne pepper in a medium bowl. Add the shrimp to the bowl and toss to coat well.

2. Cover the bowl with plastic wrap and marinate in the refrigerator for 30 minutes.

3. Spritz the air fry basket with cooking spray. Place the shrimp in the pan and spray with cooking spray.

4. Place the basket on the air fry position.

5. Select Air Fry, set temperature to 400ºF (205ºC), and set time to 12 minutes. Flip the shrimp halfway through the cooking time.

6. When cooked, the shrimp should be opaque and crisp. Remove from the air fryer grill and serve hot.

76. Easy Coconut Scallops

Prep time: 10 minutes | Cook time: 12 minutes | Serves 2

$^1/_3$ cup shallots, chopped

1½ tablespoons olive oil

1½ tablespoons coconut aminos

1 tablespoon Mediterranean seasoning mix

½ tablespoon balsamic vinegar

½ teaspoon ginger, grated

1 clove garlic, chopped

1 pound (454 g) scallops, cleaned Cooking spray

Belgian endive, for garnish

1. Place all the ingredients except the scallops and Belgian endive in a small skillet over medium heat and stir to combine. Let this mixture simmer for about 2 minutes.

2. Remove the mixture from the skillet to a large bowl and set aside to cool.

3. Add the scallops, coating them all over, then transfer to the refrigerator to marinate for at least 2 hours.

4. When ready, place the scallops in the air fry basket in a single layer and spray with cooking spray.

5. Place the basket on the air fry position.

6. Select Air Fry, set temperature to 345ºF (174ºC), and set time to 10 minutes. Flip the scallops halfway through the cooking time.

7. When cooking is complete, the scallops should be tender and opaque. Remove from the air fryer grill and serve garnished with the Belgian endive.

77. Breaded Crab Sticks with Mayo Sauce

Prep time: 5 minutes | Cook time: 12 minutes | Serves 4
Crab Sticks:

2 eggs

1 cup flour

$^1/_3$ cup panko bread crumbs

1 tablespoon old bay seasoning

1 pound (454 g) crab sticks

Cooking spray

Mayo Sauce:

½ cup mayonnaise

1 lime, juiced

2 garlic cloves, minced

1. In a bowl, beat the eggs. In a shallow bowl, place the flour. In another shallow bowl, thoroughly combine the panko bread crumbs and old bay seasoning.

2. Dredge the crab sticks in the flour, shaking off any excess, then in the beaten eggs, finally press them in the bread crumb mixture to coat well.

3. Arrange the crab sticks in the air fry basket and spray with cooking spray.

4. Place the basket on the air fry position.

5. Select Air Fry, set temperature to 390ºF (199ºC), and set time to 12 minutes. Flip the crab sticks halfway through the cooking time.

6. Meanwhile, make the sauce by whisking together the mayo, lime juice, and garlic in a small bowl.

7. When cooking is complete, remove the basket from the air fryer grill. Serve the crab sticks with the mayo sauce on the side.

78. Butter-Wine Baked Salmon Steak

Prep time: 5 minutes | Cook time: 10 minutes | Serves 4

4 tablespoons butter, melted

2 cloves garlic, minced

Sea salt and ground black pepper, to taste

¼ cup dry white wine

1 tablespoon lime juice

1 teaspoon smoked paprika

½ teaspoon onion powder

4 salmon steaks

Cooking spray

1. Place all the ingredients except the salmon and oil in a shallow dish and stir to mix well.

2. Add the salmon steaks, turning to coat well on both sides. Transfer the salmon to the refrigerator to marinate for 30 minutes.

3. When ready, put the salmon steaks in the air fry basket, discarding any excess marinade. Spray the salmon steaks with cooking spray.

4. Place the basket on the air fry position.

5. Select Air Fry, set temperature to 360ºF (182ºC), and set time to 10 minutes. Flip the salmon steaks halfway through.

6. When cooking is complete, remove from the air fryer grill and divide the salmon steaks among four plates. Serve warm.

79. Shrimp Spring Rolls

Prep time: 10 minutes | Cook time: 20 minutes | Serves 4

1 tablespoon olive oil
2 teaspoons minced garlic
1 cup matchstick cut carrots
2 cups finely sliced cabbage
2 (4-ounce / 113-g) cans tiny shrimp, drained
4 teaspoons soy sauce
Salt and freshly ground black pepper, to taste
16 square spring roll wrappers
Cooking spray

1.	Spray the air fry basket with cooking spray. Set aside.

2.	Heat the olive oil in a medium skillet over medium heat until it shimmers.

3.	Add the garlic to the skillet and cook for 30 seconds. Stir in the carrots and cabbage and sauté for about 5 minutes, stirring occasionally, or until the vegetables are lightly tender.

4.	Fold in the shrimp and soy sauce and sprinkle with salt and pepper, then stir to combine. Sauté for another 2 minutes, or until the moisture is evaporated. Remove from the heat and set aside to cool.

5.	Put a spring roll wrapper on a work surface and spoon 1 tablespoon of the shrimp mixture onto the lower end of the wrapper.

6.	Roll the wrapper away from you halfway, and then fold in the right and left sides, like an envelope. Continue to roll to the very end, using a little water to seal the edge. Repeat with the remaining wrappers and filling.

7.	Place the spring rolls in the air fry basket in a single layer, leaving space between each spring roll. Mist them lightly with cooking spray.

8.	Place the basket on the air fry position.

9.	Select Air Fry, set temperature to 375ºF (190ºC), and set time to 10 minutes. Flip the rolls halfway through the cooking time.

10.	When cooking is complete, the spring rolls will be heated through and start to brown. If necessary, continue cooking for 5 minutes more. Remove from the air fryer grill and cool for a few minutes before serving.

CHAPTER 3 MAINS

80. Marinara Sauce

Prep time: 15 minutes | Cook time: 30 minutes | Makes about 3 cups

¼ cup extra-virgin olive oil

3 garlic cloves, minced

1 small onion, chopped (about ½ cup)

2 tablespoons minced or puréed sun-dried tomatoes (optional)

1 (28-ounce / 794-g) can crushed tomatoes

½ teaspoon dried basil

½ teaspoon dried oregano

¼ teaspoon red pepper flakes

1 teaspoon kosher salt or ½ teaspoon fine salt, plus more as needed

1.   Heat the oil in a medium saucepan over medium heat.

2.   Add the garlic and onion and sauté for 2 to 3 minutes, or until the onion is softened. Add the sun-dried tomatoes (if desired) and cook for 1 minute until fragrant. Stir in the crushed tomatoes, scraping any brown bits from the bottom of the pot. Fold in the basil, oregano, red pepper flakes, and salt. Stir well.

3.   Bring to a simmer. Cook covered for about 30 minutes, stirring occasionally.

4.   Turn off the heat and allow the sauce to cool for about 10 minutes.

5.   Taste and adjust the seasoning, adding more salt if needed.

6.   Use immediately.

81. Spicy Southwest Seasoning

Prep time: 5 minutes | Cook time: 0 minutes | Makes about ¾ cups

1 tablespoon granulated onion

1 tablespoon granulated garlic

2 tablespoons dried oregano

2 tablespoons freshly ground black pepper

3 tablespoons ancho chile powder

3 tablespoons paprika

2 teaspoons cayenne

2 teaspoons cumin

1.   Stir together all the ingredients in a small bowl.

2.   Use immediately or place in an airtight container in the pantry.

82. .Classic Caesar Salad Dressing

Prep time: 5 minutes | Cook time: 0 minutes | Makes about ⅔ cup

½ cup extra-virgin olive oil

1 teaspoon anchovy paste

2 tablespoons freshly squeezed lemon juice

¼ teaspoon kosher salt or ⅛ teaspoon fine salt

¼ teaspoon minced or pressed garlic

1 egg, beaten

1.   Add all the ingredients to a tall, narrow container.

2.   Purée the mixture with an immersion blender until smooth.

3.   Use immediately.

83. Baked White Rice

Prep time: 3 minutes | Cook time: 35 minutes | Makes about 4 cups

1 cup long-grain white rice, rinsed and drained

2 cups water

1 tablespoon unsalted butter, melted, or 1 tablespoon extra-virgin olive oil

1 teaspoon kosher salt or ½ teaspoon fine salt

1.   Add the butter and rice to the baking pan and stir to coat. Pour in the water and sprinkle with the salt. Stir until the salt is dissolved.

2.   Place the pan on the bake position. Select Bake, set the temperature to 325ºF (163ºC), and set the time for 35 minutes.

3.   After 20 minutes, remove the pan from the air fryer grill. Stir the rice. Transfer the pan back to the air fryer grill and continue cooking for 10 to 15 minutes, or until the rice is mostly cooked through and the water is absorbed.

4.   When done, remove the pan from the air fryer grill and cover with aluminum foil. Let stand for 10 minutes. Using a fork, gently fluff the rice.

5.   Serve immediately.

84. Beef & Asparagus

Preparation Time: 40 minutes
Cooking Time: 10 minutes

Servings: 2

Ingredients:

- 2 New York strips steaks, sliced into cubes

Marinade

- 1 teaspoon olive oil
- 1 teaspoon steak seasoning
- ½ teaspoon dried onion powder
- ½ teaspoon dried garlic powder
- Salt and pepper to taste
- Pinch cayenne pepper

Asparagus

- 1 lb. asparagus
- Salt to taste
- 1 teaspoon olive oil

Method:

1. Preheat your air fryer to 400 degrees F.
2. Combine marinade ingredients in a bowl.
3. Stir in steak cubes.
4. Cover and marinate for 30 minutes.
5. Air fry at 5 minutes.
6. Coat asparagus with oil.
7. Season with salt.
8. Add asparagus to the air fryer.
9. Toss to combine.
10. Cook for another 3 to 5 minutes.

Serving Suggestions: *Garnish with chopped parsley.*

Preparation & Cooking Tips: *You can also use beef chuck for this recipe.*

85. Teriyaki Sauce

Prep time: 5 minutes | Cook time: 0 minutes | Makes ¾ cup

½ cup soy sauce

3 tablespoons honey

1 tablespoon rice wine or dry sherry

1 tablespoon rice vinegar

2 teaspoons minced fresh ginger

2 garlic cloves, smashed

1. Beat together all the ingredients in a small bowl.
2. Use immediately.

86. Roast Beef

Preparation Time: 10 minutes

Cooking Time: 30 minutes

Servings: 6

Ingredients:

- 4 lb. beef roast
- 1 tablespoon olive oil
- 1 teaspoon steak seasoning

Method:

1. Drizzle roast with oil.
2. Sprinkle with steak seasoning.
3. Add to the air fryer.
4. Select rotisserie.
5. Cook at 360 degrees F for 50 minutes.

Serving Suggestions: *Let rest for 5 minutes before serving.*

Preparation & Cooking Tips: *For well-done, final internal temperature should be 160 degrees F.*

CHAPTER 4 MEATS

87. Easy Spicy Steaks with Salad

Prep time: 15 minutes | Cook time: 15 minutes | Serves 4

1 (1½-pound / 680-g) boneless top sirloin steak, trimmed and halved crosswise

1½ teaspoons chili powder

1½ teaspoons ground cumin

¾ teaspoon ground coriander

⅛ teaspoon cayenne pepper

⅛ teaspoon ground cinnamon

1¼ teaspoons plus ⅛ teaspoon salt, divided

½ teaspoon plus ⅛ teaspoon ground black pepper, divided

1 teaspoon plus 1½ tablespoons extra-virgin olive oil, divided

3 tablespoons mayonnaise

1½ tablespoons white wine vinegar

1 tablespoon minced fresh dill

1 small garlic clove, minced

8 ounces (227 g) sugar snap peas, strings removed and cut in half on bias

½ English cucumber, halved lengthwise and sliced thin

2 radishes, trimmed, halved and sliced thin

2 cups baby arugula

1.   In a bowl, coriander, cumin, cayenne pepper, mix chili powder, cinnamon, 1¼ teaspoons salt and ½ teaspoon pepper until well combined.

2.   Add the steaks to another bowl and pat dry with paper towels. Brush with 1 teaspoon oil and transfer to the bowl of spice mixture. Roll over to coat thoroughly.

3.   Arrange the coated steaks in the air fry basket, spaced evenly apart.

4.   Place the basket on the air fry position.

5.   Select Air Fry. Set temperature to 400ºF (205ºC) and set time to 15 minutes. Flip the steak halfway through to ensure even cooking.

6.   When cooking is complete, an instant-read thermometer inserted in the thickest part of the meat should register at least 145ºF (63ºC).

7.   Transfer the steaks to a clean work surface and wrap with aluminum foil. Let stand while preparing salad.

8.   Make the salad: In a large bowl, stir together 1½ tablespoons olive oil, vinegar, mayonnaise, dill, garlic, ⅛ teaspoon pepper, and ⅛ teaspoon salt. Add snap peas, cucumber, radishes and arugula. Toss to blend well.

9.   Slice the steaks and serve with the salad.

88. Spring Rolls

Preparation Time: 15 minutes

Cooking Time: 8 minutes

Servings: 4

Ingredients:

- 8 rice paper wrappers
- 4 cups ground pork, cooked
- 2 cloves garlic, minced
- 3 scallions, chopped
- 1 tablespoon ginger, minced
- 2 cup shiitake mushrooms
- 1 cup carrot, sliced into thin strips
- 1 teaspoon sesame oil
- 3 tablespoons soy sauce
- 2 tablespoons cilantro

Method:

1.   Add rice paper wrappers on your kitchen table.

2.   Mix the remaining ingredients in a bowl.

3.   Top each of the wrappers with the ground pork mixture.

4.   Roll up the wrappers.

5.   Place in the air fryer.

6.   Choose air fry setting.

7.   Cook at 400 degrees F for 5 minutes.

8.   Turn and cook for another 3 minutes.

Serving Suggestions: ***Serve with chili dipping sauce.***

Preparation & Cooking Tips: Use lean ground pork.

89. Bacon & Broccoli Rice Bowl

Preparation Time: 10 minutes

Cooking Time: 10 minutes

Servings: 4

Ingredients:

- 8 slices bacon
- 4 cups cooked rice
- 4 cups broccoli, steamed
- 1 carrot, sliced into thin sticks

Method:

1. Add the bacon to the air fryer.
2. Set it to air fry.
3. Cook at 400 degrees F for 10 minutes or until crispy.
4. Add rice to serving bowls.
5. Top with the bacon, broccoli and carrots.

Serving Suggestions: ***Drizzle with hot sauce.***

Preparation & Cooking Tips: ***You can also roast broccoli in the air fryer if you like.***

90. Paprika Pork Chops with Corn

Preparation Time: 10 minutes
Cooking Time: 15 minutes
Servings: 4

Ingredients:

- 4 boneless pork chops
- 2 tablespoons olive oil
- 2 teaspoons paprika
- 1 teaspoon onion powder
- Salt and pepper to taste
- 4 ears corn, grilled

Method:

1. Brush both sides of pork chops with oil.
2. Season with paprika, onion powder, salt and pepper.
3. Add pork chops to the air fryer.
4. Set it to grill.
5. Cook at 375 degrees F for 5 to 7 minutes per side.
6. Serve with grilled corn.

Serving Suggestions: ***Serve with mustard.***

Preparation & Cooking Tips: Use boneless pork chops.

91. Chuck Steak and Pork Sausage Meatloaf

Prep time: 10 minutes | Cook time: 25 minutes | Serves 4

¾ pound (340 g) ground chuck
4 ounces (113 g) ground pork sausage
2 eggs, beaten
1 cup Parmesan cheese, grated
1 cup chopped shallot
3 tablespoons plain milk
1 tablespoon oyster sauce
1 tablespoon fresh parsley

1 teaspoon garlic paste
1 teaspoon chopped porcini mushrooms
½ teaspoon cumin powder
Seasoned salt and crushed red pepper flakes, to taste

1. In a large bowl, combine all the ingredients until well blended.
2. Place the meat mixture in the baking pan. Use a spatula to press the mixture to fill the pan.
3. Place the pan on the bake position.
4. Select Bake, set temperature to 360ºF (182ºC) and set time to 25 minutes.
5. When cooking is complete, the meatloaf should be well browned.
6. Let the meatloaf rest for 5 minutes.

Transfer to a serving dish and slice. Serve warm.

92. Barbecue Pork Tenderloin

Preparation Time: 10 minutes
Cooking Time: 20 minutes
Servings: 2

Ingredients:

- ½ lb. pork tenderloin, diced
- ¼ cup barbecue sauce
- 1 teaspoon olive oil

Method:

1. Coat the pork tenderloin in olive oil.
2. Brush with barbecue sauce.
3. Place in the air fryer rack.
4. Choose grill function.
5. Cook at 375 degrees F for 15 to 20 minutes.

Serving Suggestions: ***Serve with vinegar dipping sauce.***

Preparation & Cooking Tips: Use lean pork tenderloin.

93. Garlic Pork Chops with Roasted Broccoli

Preparation Time: 10 minutes
Cooking Time: 10 minutes
Servings: 2

Ingredients:

- 2 pork chops
- 2 tablespoons avocado oil, divided
- 1 teaspoon garlic powder
- ½ teaspoon paprika
- Salt to taste

- 2 cups broccoli florets
- 2 cloves garlic, minced

Method:
1. Preheat your air fryer to 350 degrees F.
2. Choose air fry setting.
3. Drizzle pork chops with half of avocado oil.
4. Season with garlic powder, paprika and salt.
5. Add to the air fryer.
6. Cook for 5 minutes.
7. Toss the broccoli in remaining oil.
8. Sprinkle with minced garlic and salt.
9. Add broccoli to the air fryer.
10. Cook for another 5 minutes.

Serving Suggestions: *Drizzle with hot sauce and serve.*

Preparation & Cooking Tips: *Use pork chops that are ½ inch thick.*

94. Pork Belly Bites

Preparation Time: 15 minutes
Cooking Time: 20 minutes
Servings: 4

Ingredients:
- 1 lb. pork belly, diced
- Salt and pepper to taste
- ½ teaspoon garlic powder
- 1 teaspoon Worcestershire sauce

Method:
1. Select the grill setting in your air fryer.
2. Preheat it to 400 degrees F.
3. Season pork with salt, pepper, garlic powder and Worcestershire sauce.
4. Add to the air fryer.
5. Cook at 400 degrees F for 20 minutes, flipping twice.

Serving Suggestions: *Serve with barbecue sauce.*
Preparation & Cooking Tips: *Add cayenne pepper if you like your pork belly bites spicy.*

95. Salt-and-Pepper Beef Roast

This meat meal will taste the most tender when it is thinly sliced.

Prep time and cooking time: 4.5 hours | Serves: 12-14

Ingredients to Use:
4-6lbs boned beef cross rib roast
1/4 cup coarse salt

1/4 cup sugar
2 tbsp. coarse-ground pepper
1/2 cup prepared horseradish

Step-by-Step Directions to cook:
1. **Mix salt with sugar in a bowl. Pat the mixture on the beef, and marinate for 3-4 hours.**
2. **Mix 1.5 tsp. salt, pepper, and horseradish.**
3. **Put the beef on a rack in a 9"x13" pan and rub the horseradish mixture.**
4. **Roast in 176$\underline{0}$C or 350$\underline{0}$F in the PowerXL Air Fryer Grill. Check if the internal temperature is 120-125$\underline{0}$C.**
5. **Rest for 20 minutes, and then slice the meat thinly across the grain.**

Nutritional Value per Serving:
Calories: 267kcal, Carbs: 1.3g, Protein: 20g, Fat: 19g.

96. Parmesan Pork Chops

Preparation Time: 10 minutes
Cooking Time: 15 minutes
Servings: 4

Ingredients:
- 4 pork chops
- 2 tablespoons olive oil
- 1 teaspoon onion powder
- 1 teaspoon garlic powder
- 1 teaspoon paprika
- ½ cup Parmesan cheese, grated
- Salt and pepper to taste

Method:
1. Brush pork chops with oil.
2. In a bowl, mix the remaining ingredients.
3. Sprinkle pork chops with spice mixture.
4. Add to the air fryer.
5. Choose grill setting.
6. Cook at 375 degrees F for 5 to 7 minutes per side.

Serving Suggestions: *Serve with marinara dipping sauce.*

Preparation & Cooking Tips: *Use bone-in pork chops for this recipe.*

97. Pork and Beef Stuffed Bell Peppers

Prep time: 20 minutes | Cook time: 18 minutes | Serves 4
¾ pound (340 g) lean ground beef

4 ounces (113 g) lean ground pork

¼ cup onion, minced

1 (15-ounce / 425-g) can crushed tomatoes

1 teaspoon Worcestershire sauce

1 teaspoon barbecue seasoning

1 teaspoon honey

½ teaspoon dried basil

½ cup cooked brown rice

½ teaspoon garlic powder

½ teaspoon oregano

½ teaspoon salt

2 small bell peppers, cut in half, stems removed, deseeded

Cooking spray

1.   Spritz a baking pan with cooking spray.

2.   Arrange the beef, pork, and onion in the baking pan.

3.   Place the pan on the bake position.

4.   Select Bake, set temperature to 360ºF (182ºC) and set time to 8 minutes. Break the ground meat into chunks halfway through the cooking.

5.   When cooking is complete, the ground meat should be lightly browned.

6.   Meanwhile, combine the tomatoes, honey, barbecue seasoning, Worcestershire sauce, and basil in a saucepan. Stir to mix well.

7.   Transfer the cooked meat mixture to a large bowl and add the cooked rice, garlic powder, salt, oregano, and ¼ cup of the tomato mixture. Stir to mix well.

8.   Stuff the pepper halves with the mixture, then arrange the pepper halves in the air fry basket.

9.   Select Air Fry. Set time to 10 minutes. Place the basket on the air fry position.

10.   When cooking is complete, the peppers should be lightly charred.

11.   Serve the stuffed peppers with the remaining tomato sauce on top.

98.   Mustard Herbed Pork Chops

Preparation Time: 40 minutes

Cooking Time: 20 minutes

Servings: 4

Ingredients:

- 2 teaspoons Dijon mustard
- 4 teaspoons white wine
- 4 teaspoons olive oil

- 4 pork chops
- 1 teaspoon dried rosemary leaves
- 1 teaspoon ground coriander
- 1 clove garlic, minced
- Salt and pepper to taste

Method:

1.   Mix mustard, wine and oil in a bowl.

2.   Add pork chops and marinate for 30 minutes.

3.   Sprinkle with rosemary, coriander, garlic, salt and pepper.

4.   Choose grill setting in the air fryer.

5.   Preheat it to 350 degrees F.

6.   Add pork chops to the air fryer.

7.   Cook for 10 minutes per side.

Serving Suggestions: *Let pork chops rest for 5 minutes before serving.*

Preparation & Cooking Tips: *Use pork chops that are ¾ inch thick.*

99.   Pork Chops with Creamy Dip

Preparation Time: 10 minutes

Cooking Time: 30 minutes

Servings: 4

Ingredients:

Sauce

- 3 tablespoons mayonnaise
- 1 teaspoon apple cider vinegar
- 1 tablespoon honey
- 1 tablespoon mustard
- ¼ teaspoon paprika
- Salt and pepper to taste

Pork

- 4 pork chops
- Salt and pepper to taste
- ¼ cup all-purpose flour
- 2 eggs
- ¾ cup breadcrumbs

Method:

1.   In a bowl, mix the ingredients for sauce.

2.   Refrigerate until serving time.

3.   Season pork chops with salt and pepper.

4.   Coat with flour.

5.   Dip in eggs and dredge with breadcrumbs.

6.   Press air fry setting.

7. Cook at 360 degrees F for 30 minutes, flipping once.

8. Serve pork chops with dip.

Serving Suggestions: **Serve with fresh green salad.**
Preparation & Cooking Tips: Use Dijon mustard.

100.Perfect Air Fryer Pork Chops

Prep/Cook Time 35 minutes, Servings 4 people
Ingredients

- 4 thick cut pork chops
- 2 tsp sage
- 2 tsp thyme
- 2 tsp oregano
- 1 tsp rosemary
- 1 tsp paprika
- 1 tsp garlic powder
- 1 tsp salt
- 1/2 tsp black pepper

Instructions

- Combine the sage, thyme, oregano, rosemary, paprika, garlic powder, salt, and black pepper. Set aside.
- Preheat your Air Fryer to 360 degrees Fahrenheit.
- While you Air Fryer is preheating, rub a little bit of olive oil over the pork chops and sprinkle the herb mixture over the chops, covering all sides.
- Place in Air Fryer basket making sure the chops don't overlap.
- Cook on 360 degrees for 14-16 minutes, flipping halfway. Pork chops are done when they have reached an internal temperature of 145 degrees Fahrenheit.
- Remove pork chops from the Air Fryer and loosely cover with foil. Allow them to rest for about 5 minutes.

Nutrition Info : Calories: 217kcal, Carbohydrates: 2g, Protein: 29g, Fat: 10g, Saturated Fat: 3g, Cholesterol: 90mg, Sodium: 647mg, Potassium: 522mg, Fiber: 1g, Sugar: 1g

101.Perfect Rump Roast

Rump roast makes for a wonderful Sunday dinner meal.
Prep time and cooking time: 2 hours | Serves: 5
Ingredients to Use:

4lb rump roast
3 Garlic cloves
1 tbsp. each of salt, pepper
1 onion
1 cup water
Step-by-Step Directions to Cook:
1. *Preheat the PowerXL Air Fryer Grill to 260ºC or 500ºF*
2. *Make 4-5 cuts on the roast, and fill with salt, pepper, and garlic.*
3. *Season some more before searing for 20 mins. Add water and minced onion.*
4. *Cook in the PowerXL Air Fryer Grill at 180ºC or 350ºF for 1.5 hours.*
Nutritional Value per Serving:
Calories: 916.8kcal, Carbs: 4.4g, Protein: 94.6g, Fat: 55.2g.

102.Air Fryer Juicy Steak Fasteat

Prep/Cook Time: 20 minutes, Servings: 1 person
Ingredients

- 250 g Steak - 1-1.5 in/2.5-3.5 cm thick - Top Sirloin or New York strip or Filet Mignon or a ribeye or any other favourite cut
- Salt - to taste
- Black pepper - to taste freshly ground
- 1 tsp Olive oil - optional - or butter

Instructions

- Bring the steak to room temperature** (this helps it cook more evenly as the heat penetrates much easier when the meat is not frozen).
- Preheat your air fryer for 3 minutes or until 400°F (200°C).
- While you're waiting, make sure to trim any connective tissue or large pieces of fat from the edges of your steak—it should pull off easily, but you can use a sharp knife.
- Season the steak and rub it all over with olive oil. The oil is optional, but it helps crust the outside of the meat and adds extra flavour.
- Place the steak inside the air fryer basket, do not overlap the steaks. If cooking in more than two steaks, make sure not to overcrowd the Air Fryer basket. If needed, cook in batches to avoid overcrowding. The first batch will take longer to cook if Air Fryer is not already pre-heated.

- If there is a temperature setting (mine doesn't), set the temperature to 400°F (200°C).
- Cook for 6-18 minutes, flipping halfway through cooking. Cooking time depends on how thick and cold the steaks are plus how done you prefer your steaks. You can adjust cooking times to your preferred doneness. Use a quick read thermometer to check the internal temperature of the meat. It is the safest way to know that the steak is cooked to your desired doneness.
- Remove it from the air fryer, and let it rest for about 5-10 minutes before slicing.
- Serve immediately.

Nutrition Info
Calories: 560kcal, Protein: 50g, Fat: 40g, Saturated Fat: 16g, Cholesterol: 153mg, Sodium: 130mg, Potassium: 670mg, Calcium: 18mg, Iron: 4.3mg

103.Air Fryer Jerk Steak with Compound Butter

Prep/Cook Time: 15 minutes, Servings: 1 people
Ingredients
- 8 oz ribeye steak
- 1/2 tbsp jerk spice
- 1 tbsp compound butter
- 1 tbsp olive oil

Instructions
- Brush steak with olive oil. Rub steak with jerk seasoning
- Preheat air fryer to 400 degrees F.
- Add steak and fry for 10-14 minutes, flipping halfway
- Remove steak and let rest 5-10 minutes. Top with butter. Serve

Nutrition Info
Calories: 707kcal, Carbohydrates: 2g, Protein: 46g, Fat: 58g, Saturated Fat: 23g, Cholesterol: 168mg

104.Air Fryer Bacon Wrapped Beef Tenderloin

Prep/Cook Time: 25 Min Servings: 4
Ingredients
- 4 (5 oz.) bacon wrapped beef tenderloins
- Salt and pepper for seasoning

Instructions

- Season both sides of the tenderloins with salt and pepper. Place tenderloins in the bowl.
- Tap the grill button and set temperature to 425°F and fry for 16-20 minutes, turning tenderloins halfway through.
- Remove the tenderloins and place on a cutting board to rest for 5-10 minutes.
- Serve tenderloins with steak sauce and your favorite steamed vegetable.

Nutrition Info
Calories 352 Calories from Fat 99, Fat 10g, Saturated Fat 6g, Cholesterol 80mg, Sodium 821mg, Protein 27g

105.Slow Roasted Beef Short Ribs

Beef short ribs always taste delicious with this recipe. Prep time and cooking time: 3 hours 10 minutes | Serves: 6
Ingredients to Use:
5lbs beef short ribs
1/3 cup brown sugar
1 tsp. garlic powder
1 tsp. onion powder
1/4 tsp. marjoram
1/2 tsp. kosher salt
1/4 tsp. thyme
1 pinch cayenne pepper
Step-by-Step Directions to cook:
1. *Pat the ribs dry.*
2. *Rub the ingredients on each rib, put them in a sealed plastic bag, and freeze overnight.*
3. *Preheat the PowerXL Air Fryer Grill to 150ᴏC or 300ᴏF, and put ribs on a rack in a roasting pan.*
4. *Roast for around 3 hours.*
Nutritional Value per Serving:
Calories: 791kcal, Carbs: 19g, Protein: 79g, Fat: 42g.

106.Air Fryer BBQ Pork Tenderloin

Prep/Cook Time: 20 minutes, Servings: 2 people
Ingredients
- 285 grams Pork Tenderloin
- 1/4 cup BBQ Sauce
- 1 tsp Olive Oil

Instructions
- Pat the pork tenderloin dry then dice them.

- Toss the pork tenderloin in olive oil and barbecue sauce to coat.
- Place pork tenderloin in the air fryer basket with no crowding and overlapping.
- Air Fry for 15 minutes at 375F (190C)

Nutrition Info
Calories: 290, Total Fat: 8g, Saturated Fat: 2g, Sodium: 444mg, Carbohydrates: 14g, Sugar: 12g, Protein: 37g

107.Air Fried Masala Chops

Prep/Cook Time: 37 minutes, Servings: 4

Ingredients
- Lamb/Goat chops 500 g
- Kashmiri red chili powder 1-1/2 tbsp
- Turmeric powder 1 tbsp
- Garam Masala Powder 1/2 tbsp
- Salt 1 tsp
- Cumin powder 1 tbsp
- White vinegar 1 tbsp
- Ginger Garlic paste 2 tbsp
- Oil 2-3 tbsp

Instructions
- Heat 2-3 tbsp oil in pan/wok.
- Add 2 tbsp ginger garlic paste. Stir few seconds, do not burn it.
- Add chops, cook until colour change and all extra juices from meat evaporate.
- Now add all remaining ingredients from above list with some water and stir few seconds.
- Add 1/2 cup water and cook for 25 minutes almost.
- Turn the heat high and dry it.
- Now keep these chops in air fryer and cook at 180 C for 8-10 minutes.
- Done. Serve with any yogurt dip you like.

Nutrition Info
Calories 420 Calories from Fat 18, Total Fat 2g, Cholesterol 33mg, Total Carbohydrates 14g

108.London Broil Steak

A perfectly tender and flavorful meat dish.
Prep time and cooking time: 75 minutes | Serves: 6

Ingredients to Use:
2 lb. London broil top-round steak
Kosher salt
Freshly ground black pepper

1/4 cup extra-virgin olive oil
1/2 Lemon juice
2 tbsp. brown sugar
1 tbsp. Worcestershire sauce
4 cloves garlic, diced
1/4 cup Balsamic vinegar

Step-by-Step Directions to cook:
1. *Marinate the steak in the refrigerator for at least 20 mins.*
2. *Preheat the PowerXL Air Fryer Grill to 190OC or 375OF, and cook the steak for 6-8 mins on each side.*

Nutritional Value per Serving:
Calories: 173kcal, Protein: 26.1g, Fat: 7.7g.

109.Air Fryer Marinated Steak

Prep/Cook Time 15 minutes, Servings 2

Ingredients
- 2 Butcher Box New York Strip Steaks (mine were about 6-8 oz each) You can use any cut of steak
- 1 tablespoon low-sodium soy sauce This is used to provide liquid to marinate the meat and make it juicy.
- 1 teaspoon liquid smoke or a cap full
- 1 tablespoon McCormick's Grill Mates Montreal Steak Seasoning or Steak Rub (or season to taste)
- 1/2 tablespoon unsweetened cocoa powder
- salt and pepper to taste
- melted butter (optional)

Instructions
- Drizzle the Butcher Box Steak with the soy sauce and liquid smoke. You can do this inside Ziploc bags.
- Season the steak with the seasonings.
- Refrigerate for at least a couple of hours, preferably overnight.
- Place the steak in the air fryer. I did not use any oil. Cook two steaks at a time (if air fryer is standard size). You can use an accessory grill pan, a layer rack or the standard air fryer basket.
- Cook for 5 minutes on 370 degrees. After 5 minutes, open the air fryer and examine your steak. Cook time will vary depending on your desired doneness. Use a meat thermometer and cook to 125° F for rare, 135° F for medium-rare, 145° F for

medium, 155° F for medium-well, and 160° F for well done.

- I cooked the steak for an additional 2 minutes for medium-done steak.
- Remove the steak from the air fryer and drizzle with melted butter.

Nutrition Info

Calories 476kcal, Total Fat: 2g, Carbohydrates: 2g Protein: 17g

110.Air Fryer Pork Belly Bites

Prep/Cook Time: 30 mins, Servings: 4 servings

Ingredients

- 1 lb. pork belly , rinsed & patted dry
- 1 teaspoon Worcestershire sauce or soy sauce
- 1/2 teaspoon garlic powder
- salt , to taste
- black pepper , to taste
- 1/4 cup BBQ sauce (optional)

Instructions

- Preheat the Air Fryer at 400°F for 4 minutes. This will give the pork bites a really good sear.
- If needed, remove the skin from the pork belly. Cut the pork belly into 3/4"◻ sized cubes and place in a bowl. Season with Worcestershire sauce, garlic powder, salt and pepper. Spread the pork belly in even layer in air fryer basket.
- Air Fry at 400°F for 10-18 minutes, shaking and flipping and the pork belly 2 times through cooking process (time depends on your preferred doneness, thickness of the pork belly, size & cooking intensity of your air fryer).
- If you want it more done, add an extra 2-5 minutes of cooking time. Check the pork belly to see how well done it is cooked.
- Season with additional salt & pepper if desired. It needs a good amount of seasoning to bring out the flavors. Drizzle with optional bbq sauce if desired. Serve warm.

Nutrition Info

Calories: 590kcal, Carbohydrates: 1g, Protein: 11g, Fat: 60g, Saturated Fat: 22g, Cholesterol: 82mg, Sodium: 342mg, Potassium: 222mg, Sugar: 1g, Vitamin C: 0.3mg, Calcium: 6mg, Iron: 0.7mg

111.Breaded Boneless Pork Chops with Creamy Dipping Sauce

Prep/Cook Time: 20 min, Servings: 4 people

Ingredients

Sauce

- 3 TBS good mayonnaise
- 1 TBS Dijon mustard
- 1 TBS honey
- 1 tsp apple cider vinegar
- 1/2 tsp sea salt
- 1/4 tsp freshly ground pepper
- 1/4 tsp paprika

Pork

- 4 (4 ounce) boneless pork chops, approximately 1/2" thick
- 1/4 cup all-purpose flour
- 1/2 tsp sea salt
- 1/2 tsp freshly ground pepper
- 2 whole eggs
- 3/4 cup panko breadcrumbs
- 1 TBS parmesan cheese

Instructions:

- In a small bowl, whisk together the mayonnaise, mustard, honey, vinegar, salt, and pepper. Cover and refrigerate until ready to serve.
- Rinse the pork chops and dry them well with paper towels. Set aside.
- On one plate, place the flour and season it with salt and pepper. In a medium bowl, whisk the eggs. On another plate, place the breadcrumbs, cheese, and paprika. Mix to combine with a fork.
- Set the air fryer to 360°F and 20 minutes.
- Dip one pork chop to coat completely in the flour. Shake off the excess. Dip next into the egg wash and allow the excess egg to drip off. Then, coat the chop with the breadcrumbs. Repeat with the remaining 3 chops.
- After 5 minutes of preheating, place the chops in the fryer. You can either layer these using the wire rack, or cook in batches if they don't all fit. Cook for 10 to 15 minutes, depending on the thickness, until the internal temperature reaches approximately 150°F.
- Remove the chops to a cutting board or serving platter and allow them to rest for 5 minutes.

- Serve the pork with the dipping sauce and a green salad.

Nutrition Info
Calories: 310, Total Fat: 62gSaturated Fat: 21gTrans Fat: 1gUnsaturated Fat: 34gCholesterol: 105mg

112.Simple Lamb Chops with Horseradish Sauce

Prep time: 10 minutes | Cook time: 13 minutes | Serves 4

For the Lamb:

4 lamb loin chops

2 tablespoons vegetable oil

1 clove garlic, minced

½ teaspoon kosher salt

½ teaspoon black pepper

For the Horseradish Cream Sauce:

1 to 1½ tablespoons prepared horseradish

1 tablespoon Dijon mustard

½ cup mayonnaise

2 teaspoons sugar

Cooking spray

1. Spritz the air fry basket with cooking spray.
2. Place the lamb chops on a plate. Rub with the sprinkle and oil with the garlic, salt and black pepper. Let sit to marinate for 30 minutes at room temperature.
3. Make the horseradish cream sauce: Mix the horseradish, mayonnaise, mustard, and sugar in a bowl until well combined. Set half of the sauce aside until ready to serve.
4. Arrange the marinated chops in the air fry basket.
5. Place the basket on the air fry position.
6. Select Air Fry. Set temperature to 325ºF (163ºC) and set time to 10 minutes. Flip the lamb chops halfway through.
7. When cooking is complete, the lamb should be lightly browned.
8. Transfer the chops from the air fryer grill to the bowl of the horseradish sauce. Roll to coat well.
9. Put the coated chops back in the air fry basket on the air fry position. Select Air Fry. Set the temperature to 400ºF (205ºC) and the time to 3 minutes.
10. When cooking is complete, the internal temperature should reach 145ºF (63ºC) on a meat thermometer (for medium-rare). Flip the lamb halfway through.
11. Serve hot with the horseradish cream sauce.

113.Easy Cinnamon Steak

Prep time: 10 minutes | Cook time: 13 minutes | Makes 12 koftas

1½ pounds (680 g) lean ground beef

1 teaspoon onion powder

¾ teaspoon ground cinnamon

¾ teaspoon ground dried turmeric

1 teaspoon ground cumin

¾ teaspoon salt

¼ teaspoon cayenne

12 (3½- to 4-inch-long) cinnamon sticks

Cooking spray

1. Spritz the air fry basket with cooking spray.
2. Combine all the ingredients, except for the cinnamon sticks, in a large bowl. Toss to mix well.
3. Divide and shape the mixture into 12 balls, then wrap each ball around each cinnamon stick and leave a quarter of the length uncovered.
4. Arrange the beef-cinnamon sticks in the prepared basket and spritz with cooking spray.
5. Place the basket on the air fry position.
6. Select Air Fry. Set temperature to 375ºF (190ºC) and set time to 13 minutes. Flip the sticks halfway through the cooking.
7. When cooking is complete, the beef should be browned.
8. Serve immediately.

114.Air Fryer Carne Asada Recipe

Prep/Cook Time: 26 minutes, Servings: 4 people

Ingredients
- 2 pounds Skirt Steak 1/2 thick or more
- 1 large Yellow/Brown Onion thinly sliced

Marinade
- 4-5 whole Chipotle Peppers in Adobo (from a can)
- 2 Pasilla Peppers
- 1/2 cup Freshly Squeezed Orange Juice
- 1/4 cup Freshly Squeezed Lime Juice
- 1/4 cup Freshly Squeeze Lemon Juice
- 6 cloves Fresh Garlic
- 2 Tablespoons Extra Virgin Olive Oil

- 1 cup Fresh Cilantro Leaves
- 2 Tablespoons Light Brown Sugar
- 1 Tablespoon Kosher Salt
- 2 teaspoons Ground Cumin
- 2 teaspoons Dried Oregano
- 1 teaspoon Freshly Ground Black Pepper

Instructions

- Prepare Pasilla Peppers, following this Charring Instructions.
- Add Peppers and all Marinade ingredients to food processor. Process until well blended, about 20 seconds. Hold back 1/2 cup of Marinade to use as Salsa.
- Add Marinade, Steak and Onions to a container or plastic baggie and place into refrigerator for at least three hours or overnight (which is best).
- When ready to cook, preheat Air Fryer at 400 degrees for 10 minutes.
- Remove steak from container/baggie and place into preheated Air Fryer.
- Cook at 400 degrees for 6-8 minutes (for rare), turning over after 4 minutes. Add 1-2 minutes more for medium rare.
- Remove Steak and Onions from Air Fryer and let rest for 5 minutes. Slice Steak at an angle against the grain and as thin as possible.
- Serve in Tortillas with Pico de Gallo, Avocado, Shredded Cabbage, Cilantro and Lime Wedges or use for Steak Nachos.

Nutrition Info

Calories: 254 Total Fat: 23g Saturated Fat: 11g Carbohydrates: 36g Fiber: 4g Sugar: 5g Protein: 33g

115.Panko-Crusted Lemony Schnitz e

Prep time: 15 minutes | Cook time: 15 minutes | Serves 4

4 thin boneless pork loin chops
2 tablespoons lemon juice
½ cup flour
¼ teaspoon marjoram
1 teaspoon salt
1 cup panko bread crumbs
2 eggs
Lemon wedges, for serving
Cooking spray

1. On a clean work surface, drizzle the pork chops with lemon juice on both sides.
2. Combine the flour with salt and marjoram on a shallow plate. Pour the bread crumbs on a separate shallow dish. Beat the eggs in a large bowl.
3. Dredge the pork chops in the flour, then dunk in the beaten eggs to coat well. Shake the excess off and roll over the bread crumbs. Arrange the pork chops in the air fry basket and spritz with cooking spray.
4. Place the basket on the air fry position.
5. Select Air Fry. Set temperature to 400ºF (205ºC) and set time to 15 minutes.
6. After 7 minutes, remove the basket from the air fryer grill. Flip the pork. Return the basket to the air fryer grill and continue cooking.
7. When cooking is complete, the pork should be crispy and golden.
8. Squeeze the lemon wedges over the fried chops and serve immediately.

116.Pork, Bell Pepper, and Pineapple Kebabs

Prep time: 10 minutes | Cook time: 12 minutes | Serves 4

¼ teaspoon kosher salt or ⅛ teaspoon fine salt
1 medium pork tenderloin (about 1 pound / 454 g), cut into 1½-inch chunks
1 green bell pepper, seeded and cut into 1-inch pieces
1 red bell pepper, seeded and cut into 1-inch pieces
2 cups fresh pineapple chunks
¾ cup Teriyaki Sauce or store-bought variety, divided

Special Equipment:

12 (9- to 12-inch) wooden skewers, soaked in water for about 30 minutes

1. Sprinkle the pork cubes with the salt.
2. Thread the pork, pineapple, and bell peppers onto a skewer. Repeat until all skewers are complete. Brush the skewers generously with about half of the Teriyaki Sauce. Place them on the sheet pan.
3. Place the pan on the toast position.
4. Select Toast, set temperature to 375ºF (190ºC), and set time to 10 minutes.

5. After about 5 minutes, remove the pan from the air fryer grill. Turn over the skewers and brush with the remaining half of Teriyaki Sauce. Transfer the pan back to the air fryer grill and continue cooking until the vegetables are tender and browned in places and the pork is browned and cooked through.

6. Remove the pan from the air fryer grill and serve.

117. Fast Salsa Meatballs

Prep time: 10 minutes | Cook time: 10 minutes | Serves 4

1 pound (454 g) ground beef (85% lean)
½ cup salsa
¼ cup diced green or red bell peppers
1 large egg, beaten
¼ cup chopped onions
½ teaspoon chili powder
1 clove garlic, minced
½ teaspoon ground cumin
1 teaspoon fine sea salt
Lime wedges, for serving
Cooking spray

1. Spritz the air fry basket with cooking spray.
2. Combine all the ingredients in a large bowl. Stir to mix well.
3. Divide and shape the mixture into 1-inch balls. Arrange the balls in the basket and spritz with cooking spray.
4. Place the basket on the air fry position.
5. Select Air Fry. Set temperature to 350ºF (180ºC) and set time to 10 minutes. Flip the balls with tongs halfway through.
6. When cooking is complete, the balls should be well browned.
7. Transfer the balls on a plate and squeeze the lime wedges over before serving.

118. Smoked Paprika Pork and Vegetable Kabobs

Prep time: 25 minutes | Cook time: 15 minutes | Serves 4

1 pound (454 g) pork tenderloin, cubed
1 teaspoon smoked paprika
Salt and ground black pepper, to taste
1 green bell pepper, cut into chunks
1 zucchini, cut into chunks
1 red onion, sliced
1 tablespoon oregano
Cooking spray

Special Equipment:

Small bamboo skewers, soaked in water for 20 minutes to keep them from burning while cooking

1. Spritz the air fry basket with cooking spray.
2. Add the pork to a bowl and season with the salt, black pepper, and smoked paprika. Thread the seasoned pork cubes and vegetables alternately onto the soaked skewers. Arrange the skewers in the basket.
3. Place the basket on the air fry position.
4. Select Air Fry. Set temperature to 350ºF (180ºC) and set time to 15 minutes.
5. After 7 minutes, remove the basket from the air fryer grill. Flip the pork skewers. Return the basket to the air fryer grill and continue cooking.
6. When cooking is complete, the pork should be browned and vegetables are tender.
7. Transfer the skewers to the serving dishes and sprinkle with oregano. Serve hot.

119. Fast Bacon-Wrapped Hot Dogs

Prep time: 5 minutes | Cook time: 10 minutes | Serves 5

10 thin slices of bacon
5 pork hot dogs, halved
1 teaspoon cayenne pepper

Sauce:

¼ cup mayonnaise
4 tablespoons low-carb ketchup
1 teaspoon rice vinegar
1 teaspoon chili powder

1. Arrange the slices of bacon on a clean work surface. One by one, place the halved hot dog on one end of each slice, season with cayenne pepper and wrap the hot dog with the bacon slices and secure with toothpicks as needed.
2. Place wrapped hot dogs in the air fry basket.
3. Place the basket on the air fry position.
4. Select Air Fry. Set temperature to 390ºF (199ºC) and set time to 10 minutes. Flip the bacon-wrapped hot dogs halfway through.
5. When cooking is complete, the bacon should be crispy and browned.

6. Make the sauce: Stir all the ingredients for the sauce in a small bowl. Wrap the bowl in plastic and set in the refrigerator until ready to serve.

7. Transfer the hot dogs to a platter and serve hot with the sauce.

120.Tangy Pork Ribs

Prep time: 1 hour 10 minutes | Cook time: 25 minutes | Serves 6

2½ pounds (1.1 kg) boneless country-style pork ribs, cut into 2-inch pieces
3 tablespoons olive brine
1 tablespoon minced fresh oregano leaves
$^1/_3$ cup orange juice
1 teaspoon ground cumin
1 tablespoon minced garlic
1 teaspoon salt
1 teaspoon ground black pepper
Cooking spray

1. Combine all the ingredients in a large bowl. Toss to coat the pork ribs well. Wrap the bowl in plastic and refrigerate for at least an hour to marinate.

2. Spritz the air fry basket with cooking spray.

3. Arrange the marinated pork ribs in the basket and spritz with cooking spray.

4. Place the basket on the air fry position.

5. Select Air Fry. Set temperature to 400ºF (205ºC) and set time to 25 minutes. Flip the ribs halfway through.

6. When cooking is complete, the ribs should be well browned.

7. Serve immediately.

121..Breaded Calf's Liver Strips

Prep time: 15 minutes | Cook time: 5 minutes | Serves 4

1 pound (454 g) sliced calf's liver, cut into ½-inch wide strips
2 eggs
2 tablespoons milk
½ cup whole wheat flour
2 cups panko bread crumbs
Salt and ground black pepper, to taste
Cooking spray

1. Spritz the air fry basket with cooking spray.

2. Rub the calf's liver strips with ground black pepper and salt on a clean work surface.

3. Whisk the eggs with milk in a large bowl. Pour the flour in a shallow dish. Pour the panko on a separate shallow dish.

4. Dunk the liver strips in the flour, then in the egg mixture. Shake the excess off and roll the strips over the panko to coat well.

5. Arrange the liver strips in the basket and spritz with cooking spray.

6. Place the basket on the air fry position.

7. Select Air Fry. Set temperature to 390ºF (199ºC) and set time to 5 minutes. Flip the strips halfway through.

8. When cooking is complete, the strips should be browned.

9. Serve immediately.

122..Golden Pork Tenderloin

Prep time: 5 minutes | Cook time: 10 minutes | Serves 6

2 large egg whites
1½ tablespoons Dijon mustard
2 cups crushed pretzel crumbs
1½ pounds (680 g) pork tenderloin, cut into ¼-pound (113-g) sections
Cooking spray

1. Spritz the air fry basket with cooking spray.

2. Whisk the egg whites with Dijon mustard in a bowl until bubbly. Pour the pretzel crumbs in a separate bowl.

3. Dredge the pork tenderloin in the egg white mixture and press to coat. Shake the excess off and roll the tenderloin over the pretzel crumbs.

4. Arrange the well-coated pork tenderloin in the basket and spritz with cooking spray.

5. Place the basket on the air fry position.

6. Select Air Fry. Set temperature to 350ºF (180ºC) and set time to 10 minutes.

7. After 5 minutes, remove the basket from the air fryer grill. Flip the pork. Return the basket to the air fryer grill and continue cooking.

8. When cooking is complete, the pork should be golden brown and crispy.

9. Serve immediately.

123..North African Lamb Kofta

Prep time: 25 minutes | Cook time: 10 minutes | Serves 4

1 pound (454 g) ground lamb
1 tablespoon ras el hanout (North African spice)
½ teaspoon ground coriander
1 teaspoon onion powder
1 teaspoon garlic powder
1 teaspoon cumin
2 tablespoons mint, chopped
Salt and ground black pepper, to taste

Special Equipment:

4 bamboo skewers

1.   Combine the ground lamb, ras el hanout, coriander, cumin, mint, garlic powder, onion powder, salt, and ground black pepper in a large bowl. Stir to mix well.
2.   Transfer the mixture into sausage molds and sit the bamboo skewers in the mixture. Refrigerate for 15 minutes.
3.   Spritz the air fry basket with cooking spray. Place the lamb skewers in the pan and spritz with cooking spray.
4.   Place the basket on the air fry position.
5.   Select Air Fry. Set temperature to 380ºF (193ºC) and set time to 10 minutes. Flip the lamb skewers halfway through.
6.   When cooking is complete, the lamb should be well browned.
7.   Serve immediately.

124. Panko-Crusted Wasabi Spam

Prep time: 5 minutes | Cook time: 12 minutes | Serves 3

$^2/_3$ cup all-purpose flour
2 large eggs
1½ tablespoons wasabi paste
2 cups panko bread crumbs
6 ½-inch-thick spam slices
Cooking spray

1.   Spritz the air fry basket with cooking spray.
2.   Pour the flour in a shallow plate. Whisk the eggs with wasabi in a large bowl. Pour the panko in a separate shallow plate.
3.   Dredge the spam slices in the flour first, then dunk in the egg mixture, and then roll the spam over the panko to coat well. Shake the excess off.

4.   Arrange the spam slices in the basket and spritz with cooking spray.
5.   Place the basket on the air fry position.
6.   Select Air Fry. Set temperature to 400ºF (205ºC) and set time to 12 minutes. Flip the spam slices halfway through.
7.   When cooking is complete, the spam slices should be golden and crispy.
8.   Serve immediately.

125. Golden Asparagus and Prosciutto Tart

Prep time: 10 minutes | Cook time: 25 minutes | Serves 4

All-purpose flour, for dusting
1 sheet (½ package) frozen puff pastry, thawed
½ cup grated Parmesan cheese
1 pound (454 g) (or more) asparagus, trimmed
8 ounces (227 g) thinly sliced prosciutto, sliced into ribbons about ½-inch wide
2 teaspoons aged balsamic vinegar

1.   On a lightly floured cutting board, unwrap and unfold the puff pastry and roll it lightly with a rolling pin so as to press the folds together. Place it on the sheet pan.
2.   Roll about ½ inch of the pastry edges up to form a ridge around the perimeter. Crimp the corners together to create a solid rim around the pastry. Using a fork, pierce the bottom of the pastry all over. Scatter the cheese over the bottom of the pastry.
3.   Arrange the asparagus spears on top of the cheese in a single layer with 4 or 5 spears pointing one way, the next few pointing the opposite direction. You may need to trim them so they fit within the border of the pastry shell. Lay the prosciutto on top more or less evenly.
4.   Place the pan on the bake position.
5.   Select Bake, set temperature to 375ºF (190ºC), and set time to 25 minutes.
6.   After about 15 minutes, check the tart, rotating the pan if the crust is not browning evenly and continue cooking until the pastry is golden brown and the edges of the prosciutto pieces are browned.

7. Remove the pan from the air fryer grill. Allow to cool for 5 minutes before slicing.

8. Drizzle with the balsamic vinegar just before serving.

126.Pork Butt with Garlicky Sauce

Prep time: 1 hour 15 minutes | Cook time: 30 minutes | Serves 4

1 teaspoon golden flaxseeds meal
1 egg white, well whisked
1 tablespoon soy sauce
1 teaspoon lemon juice, preferably freshly squeezed
1 tablespoon olive oil
1 pound (454 g) pork butt, cut into pieces 2-inches long
Salt and ground black pepper, to taste
Garlicky Coriander-Parsley Sauce:
3 garlic cloves, minced
$^1/_3$ cup fresh coriander leaves
$^1/_3$ cup fresh parsley leaves
1 teaspoon lemon juice
½ tablespoon salt
$^1/_3$ cup extra-virgin olive oil

1. Combine the flaxseeds meal, egg white, lemon juice, soy sauce, olive oil, salt, and black pepper in a large bowl. Dunk the pork strips in and press to submerge.

2. Wrap the bowl in plastic and refrigerate to marinate for at least an hour.

3. Arrange the marinated pork strips in the air fry basket.

4. Place the basket on the air fry position.

5. Select Air Fry. Set temperature to 380ºF (193ºC) and set time to 30 minutes.

6. After 15 minutes, remove the basket from the air fryer grill. Flip the pork. Return the basket to the air fryer grill and continue cooking.

7. When cooking is complete, the pork should be well browned.

8. Meanwhile, combine the ingredients for the sauce in a small bowl. Stir to mix well. Arrange the bowl in the refrigerator to chill until ready to serve.

9. Serve the air fried pork strips with the chilled sauce.

127.Apple-Glazed Pork Chops

Prep time: 15 minutes | Cook time: 19 minutes | Serves 4

1 sliced apple
1 small onion, sliced
2 tablespoons apple cider vinegar, divided
½ teaspoon thyme
½ teaspoon rosemary
¼ teaspoon brown sugar
3 tablespoons olive oil, divided
¼ teaspoon smoked paprika
4 pork chops
Salt and ground black pepper, to taste

1. Combine the apple slices, onion, thyme, rosemary, brown sugar, 1 tablespoon of vinegar, and 2 tablespoons of olive oil in a baking pan. Stir to mix well.

2. Place the pan on the bake position.

3. Select Bake, set temperature to 350ºF (180ºC) and set time to 4 minutes. Stir the mixture halfway through.

4. Meanwhile, combine the remaining vinegar and olive oil, and paprika in a large bowl. Sprinkle with salt and ground black pepper. Stir to mix well. Dredge the pork in the mixture and toss to coat well. Place the pork in the air fry basket.

5. When cooking is complete, remove the baking pan from the air fryer grill and place in the air fry basket.

6. Select Air Fry and set time to 10 minutes. Place the basket on the air fry position. Flip the pork chops halfway through.

7. When cooking is complete, the pork should be lightly browned.

8. Remove the pork from the air fryer grill and baste with baked apple mixture on both sides. Put the pork back to the air fryer grill and air fry for an additional 5 minutes. Flip halfway through.

9. Serve immediately.

128.Turkish Spicy Lamb Pizza

Prep time: 20 minutes | Cook time: 10 minutes | Serves 4

4 (6-inch) flour tortillas
For the Meat Topping:

4 ounces (113 g) ground lamb or 85% lean ground beef

¼ cup finely chopped green bell pepper

¼ cup chopped fresh parsley

1 small plum tomato, deseeded and chopped

2 tablespoons chopped yellow onion

1 garlic clove, minced

2 teaspoons tomato paste

¼ teaspoon sweet paprika

¼ teaspoon ground cumin

⅛ to ¼ teaspoon red pepper flakes

⅛ teaspoon ground allspice

⅛ teaspoon kosher salt

⅛ teaspoon black pepper

For Serving:

¼ cup chopped fresh mint

1 teaspoon extra-virgin olive oil

1 lemon, cut into wedges

1. Combine all the ingredients for the meat topping in a medium bowl until well mixed.

2. Lay the tortillas on a clean work surface. Spoon the meat mixture on the tortillas and spread all over.

3. Place the tortillas in the air fry basket.

4. Place the basket on the air fry position.

5. Select Air Fry. Set temperature to 400ºF (205ºC) and set time to 10 minutes.

6. When cooking is complete, the edge of the tortilla should be golden and the meat should be lightly browned.

7. Transfer them to a serving dish. Top with chopped fresh mint and drizzle with olive oil. Squeeze the lemon wedges on top and serve.

129.Panko-Crusted Beef Meatballs

Prep time: 5 minutes | Cook time: 8 minutes | Serves 4

1 pound (454 g) lean ground sirloin beef

2 tablespoons seasoned bread crumbs

¼ teaspoon kosher salt

1 large egg, beaten

1 cup marinara sauce, for serving

Cooking spray

1. Spritz the air fry basket with cooking spray.

2. Mix all the ingredients, except for the marinara sauce, into a bowl until well blended. Shape the mixture into sixteen meatballs.

3. Arrange the meatballs in the prepared basket and mist with cooking spray.

4. Place the basket on the air fry position.

5. Select Air Fry. Set temperature to 360ºF (182ºC) and set time to 8 minutes. Flip the meatballs halfway through.

6. When cooking is complete, the meatballs should be well browned.

7. Divide the meatballs among four plates and serve warm with the marinara sauce.

130.Cheesy Tomato Sauce Meatloaf

Prep time: 15 minutes | Cook time: 25 minutes | Serves 4

1½ pounds (680 g) ground beef

1 cup tomato sauce

½ cup bread crumbs

2 egg whites

½ cup grated Parmesan cheese

1 diced onion

2 tablespoons chopped parsley

2 tablespoons minced ginger

2 garlic cloves, minced

½ teaspoon dried basil

1 teaspoon cayenne pepper

Salt and ground black pepper, to taste

Cooking spray

1. Spritz a meatloaf pan with cooking spray.

2. Combine all the ingredients in a large bowl. Stir to mix well.

3. Pour the meat mixture in the prepared meatloaf pan and press with a spatula to make it firm.

4. Place the pan on the bake position.

5. Select Bake, set temperature to 360ºF (182ºC) and set time to 25 minutes.

6. When cooking is complete, the beef should be well browned.

7. Serve immediately.

131.Pork, Squash, and Pepper Kebabs

Prep time: 1 hour 20 minutes | Cook time: 8 minutes | Serves 4

For the Pork:

1 pound (454 g) pork steak, cut in cubes

1 tablespoon white wine vinegar

3 tablespoons steak sauce

¼ cup soy sauce

1 teaspoon powdered chili

1 teaspoon red chili flakes

2 teaspoons smoked paprika

1 teaspoon garlic salt

For the Vegetable:

1 green squash, deseeded and cut in cubes

1 yellow squash, deseeded and cut in cubes

1 red pepper, cut in cubes

1 green pepper, cut in cubes

Salt and ground black pepper, to taste

Cooking spray

Special Equipment:

4 bamboo skewers, soaked in water for at least 30 minutes

1.   Combine the ingredients for the pork in a large bowl. Press the pork to dunk in the marinade. Wrap the bowl in plastic and refrigerate for at least an hour.

2.   Spritz the air fry basket with cooking spray.

3.   Remove the pork from the marinade and run the skewers through the pork and vegetables alternatively. Sprinkle with salt and pepper to taste.

4.   Arrange the skewers in the pan and spritz with cooking spray.

5.   Place the basket on the air fry position.

6.   Select Air Fry. Set temperature to 380ºF (193ºC) and set time to 8 minutes.

7.   After 4 minutes, remove the basket from the air fryer grill. Flip the skewers. Return the basket to the air fryer grill and continue cooking.

8.   When cooking is complete, the pork should be browned and the vegetables should be lightly charred and tender.

9.   Serve immediately.

132.Ritzy Steak with Mushroom Gravy

Prep time: 20 minutes | Cook time: 33 minutes | Serves 2

For the Mushroom Gravy:

¾ cup sliced button mushrooms

¼ cup thinly sliced onions

¼ cup unsalted butter, melted

½ teaspoon fine sea salt

¼ cup beef broth

For the Steaks:

½ pound (227 g) ground beef (85% lean)

1 tablespoon dry mustard

2 tablespoons tomato paste

¼ teaspoon garlic powder

½ teaspoon onion powder

½ teaspoon fine sea salt

¼ teaspoon ground black pepper

Chopped fresh thyme leaves, for garnish

1.   Toss the onions and mushrooms with butter in a baking pan to coat well, then sprinkle with salt.

2.   Place the pan on the bake position.

3.   Select Bake, set temperature to 390ºF (199ºC) and set time to 8 minutes. Stir the mixture halfway through the cooking.

4.   When cooking is complete, the mushrooms should be tender.

5.   Pour the broth in the baking pan and set time to 10 more minutes to make the gravy.

6.   Meanwhile, combine all the ingredients for the steaks, except for the thyme leaves, in a large bowl. Stir to mix well. Shape the mixture into two oval steaks.

7.   Arrange the steaks over the gravy and set time to 15 minutes. When cooking is complete, the patties should be browned. Flip the steaks halfway through.

8.   Transfer the steaks onto a plate and pour the gravy over. Sprinkle with fresh thyme and serve immediately.

133.Macadamia Nuts Breaded Pork Rack

Prep time: 5 minutes | Cook time: 35 minutes | Serves 2

1 clove garlic, minced

2 tablespoons olive oil

1 pound (454 g) rack of pork

1 cup chopped macadamia nuts

1 tablespoon bread crumbs

1 tablespoon rosemary, chopped

1 egg

Salt and ground black pepper, to taste

1.   Combine the garlic and olive oil in a small bowl. Stir to mix well.

2.   On a clean work surface, rub the pork rack with the sprinkle and garlic oil with salt and black pepper on both sides.

3.   Combine the macadamia nuts, bread crumbs, and rosemary in a shallow dish. Whisk the egg in a large bowl.

4.   Dredge the pork in the egg, then roll the pork over the macadamia nut mixture to coat well. Shake the excess off.

5.   Arrange the pork in the air fry basket.

6.   Place the basket on the air fry position.

7.   Select Air Fry. Set temperature to 350ºF (180ºC) and set time to 30 minutes.

8.   After 30 minutes, remove the basket from the air fryer grill. Flip the pork rack. Return the basket to the air fryer grill and increase temperature to 390ºF (199ºC) and set time to 5 minutes. Keep cooking.

9.   When cooking is complete, the pork should be browned.

10.   Serve immediately.

CHAPTER 5 POULTRY

134. Easy Meatballs with Dijon Sauce

Prep time: 10 minutes | Cook time: 15 minutes | Serves 4

Meatballs:

½ pound (227 g) ham, diced

½ pound (227 g) ground chicken

½ cup grated Swiss cheese

1 large egg, beaten

3 cloves garlic, minced

¼ cup chopped onions

1½ teaspoons sea salt

1 teaspoon ground black pepper

Cooking spray

Dijon Sauce:

3 tablespoons Dijon mustard

2 tablespoons lemon juice

¼ cup chicken broth, warmed

¾ teaspoon sea salt

¼ teaspoon ground black pepper

Chopped fresh thyme leaves, for garnish

1.   Spritz the air fry basket with cooking spray.

2.   Combine the ingredients for the meatballs in a large bowl. Stir to mix well, then shape the mixture in twelve 1½-inch meatballs.

3.   Arrange the meatballs in the air fry basket.

4.   Place the basket on the air fry position.

5.   Select Air Fry. Set temperature to 390ºF (199ºC) and set time to 15 minutes. Flip the balls halfway through.

6.   When cooking is complete, the balls should be lightly browned.

7.   Meanwhile, combine the ingredients, except for the thyme leaves, for the sauce in a small bowl. Stir to mix well.

8.   Transfer the cooked meatballs on a large plate, then baste the sauce over. Garnish with thyme leaves and serve.

135. Easy Air Fryer Grilled Chicken

Prep/Cook Time: 25 minutes, Servings: 2-4

Ingredients

- 2–3 chicken breasts
- salt and pepper or poultry seasoning
- cooking spray

Instructions

- Preheat the air fryer to 350-360°
- Spray each side of the chicken breasts with cooking spray
- Generously season the chicken with salt and pepper or poultry seasoning
- Place in air fryer and cook for 9 minutes
- Flip the chicken over and cook for an additional 9 minutes
- Remove and serve

Nutrition Info

Calories Per Serving: 1006, Total Fat 61g, Cholesterol 300mg, Sodium 1434.1mg, Total Carbohydrate 34.9g, Sugars 27.9g, Protein 75.8g

136. Chicken Thighs with Rosemary

Roasted chicken thigh with rosemary springs and some vegetables is perfect for a great brunch.

Prep time and cooking time: 40 minutes | Serves: 4

Ingredients to use

4 chicken thighs, with the bone and skin

Rosemary sprigs

A large potato, cut into cubes

1 onion

2 tbsp. of olive oil

2 garlic cloves

Salt and pepper

1/2 tsp. of chicken seasoning powder

Step-by-Step Directions to cook it:

1.   *Preheat the PowerXL Air Fryer Grill at 218ОC or 425ОF.*

2.   *Put the rosemary sprigs on the baking pan with cooking spray.*

3.   *Bake the remaining ingredients for half an hour.*

4.   *Season the chicken thighs and bake for 35 minutes.*

Nutritional value per serving:

Calories: 670 kcal, Carbs: 14g, Protein: 47g, Fat: 46g.

137. Air Fryer Lemon Pepper Chicken

Prep/Cook Time 35 mins, Servings: 4

Ingredients

- 4 boneless-skinless chicken breasts
- 1 tbsp lemon pepper

- 1 tsp table salt
- 1-1/2 tsp granulated garlic

Instructions
- Preheat air fryer to 360 degrees for about 5 minutes.
- Sprinkle seasonings on chicken pieces.
- Place the chicken on the grill pan accessory, insert into hot air fryer & cook for 30 minutes, flipping the chicken halfway through. Internal temp should ready a min of 165 degrees.

Nutrition Info
Calories: 223kcal, Carbohydrates: 8g, Protein: 25g, Fat: 10g, Saturated Fat: 2g, Cholesterol: 59mg, Sodium: 654mg

138.Air Fryer Chicken Tenders

Prep/Cook Time: 17 minutes, Servings: 4
Ingredients
- 1 lb chicken tenderloin
- 3 eggs beaten
- 1/3 cup Panko crumbs
- 1/2 cup all-purpose flour
- 1/2 tsp salt
- 1/2 tsp pepper
- 2 Tablespoons olive oil

Instructions
- Preheat AirFryer to 330 degrees F
- Place flour, egg, and panko crumbs in three separate bowls
- Add salt, pepper, and olive oil to the Panko crumbs, mix well
- Dip chicken in the flour, then the egg, then the Panko crumbs until evenly coated
- Place in the cooking basket in the air fryer. You'll need to cook in batches.
- Fry for 12-14 minutes. Or until golden brown and internal temp reaches 165 degrees.
- Remove chicken from air fryer.
- Toss with your favorite sauce or serve with dipping sauce.

Nutrition Info
Calories 165 Fat 7g Satfat 2g Unsatfat 2g Protein 34g

139.Air Fryer General Tso's Chicken Recipe

Prep/Cook Time : 20 minutes, Servings: 2 people

Ingredients
For the Chicken
- 1 pound boneless skinless chicken thighs, cut into small pieces
- 2 tbsp cornstarch
- ½ tsp salt
- Dash of black pepper

For the Sauce
- ¼ cup ketchup
- 2 tbsp soy sauce
- 2 tbsp dark brown sugar
- ½ tsp ginger paste
- 2 garlic cloves crushed
- ½ tsp red pepper flakes

Instructions
For the Chicken
- Preheat air fryer to 400°F for 5 minutes
- In a small bowl toss the chicken with the cornstarch, salt and pepper to coat evenly
- Spray the air fryer basket with non-stick cooking spray
- Put the chicken in the air fryer, separate the pieces so they will cook all the way around
- Air fry for 10 mins, toss the basket once at 5 minutes to flip the chicken over

For the Sauce
- Add all the sauce ingredients to a small, heavy bottomed saucepan or medium heat
- Whisk until the brown sugar is dissolved
- Bring to a rapid boil
- Reduce to simmer, simmer about 5 minutes until sauce has thickened
- Pour the sauce over the air fried chicken to coat evenly
- Serve over plain white or brown rice

Nutrition Info
Calories 397 Calories from Fat 81, Fat 9g, Saturated Fat 2g, Cholesterol 215mg, Sodium 2074mg, Potassium 688mg, Carbohydrates 29g, Fiber 1g

140.Herb Roasted Turkey Breast

Moving away from the chicken recipes to another delicacy.
Prep time and cooking time: 2 hours and 40 minutes | Serves: 6
Ingredients to Use:

1/2 tsp. of minced garlic

One turkey breast, thawed

1 tsp. thyme, ground

1/2 cup of softened butter

Crushed rosemary leaves

Salt and pepper for seasoning

Step-by-Step Directions to cook it:

1.   Preheat the PowerXL Air Fryer Grill at 204̲0̲C or 400̲0̲F.

2.   Place the turkey breast on the pan after spraying cooking spray.

3.   Mix the remaining ingredients and use a brush to rub it onto the breast evenly.

4.   Roast for 2-1/2 hours and rest for 15 minutes after taking it out.

Nutritional value per serving:

Calories: 360kcal, Carbs: 1g, Protein: 72g, Fat: 5g.

141.Air Fryer Copycat Chick-fil-a Chicken Sandwich

Prep/Cook Time: 22 Minutes, 4 Servings

Ingredients

- 2 chicken boneless skinless breasts, about 12-16 Oz.
- 3/4 cup Vlassic dill pickle juice from jar
- 1 1/4 cups all purpose flour
- 2 tablespoons powdered sugar
- 1/2 teaspoon paprika
- 1/2 teaspoon salt
- 1/2 teaspoon pepper
- 1 egg
- 1/2 cup milk
- 4 hamburger buns
- fixings like tomatoes, lettuce, mayo, and pickle slices as desired

Instructions

- Filet chicken breasts in half lengthwise using a sharp knife. Pound chicken using a tenderizer until about 1/2 inch thick.
- Pour pickle juice into a bowl or plastic gallon bag, and marinate chicken for about 30 minutes or so.
- Grease air fryer basket with cooking spray or oil. I use an olive oil mister.
- Mix flour, powdered sugar, paprika, salt, and pepper in a bowl and set aside.
- Whisk together egg and milk in another bowl and set aside.
- Take the chicken out of the bag, and discard the marinade. Dip chicken in the egg mixture and then in the flour mixture. Shake a little of the flour mixture off, as you don't actually want a ton on there.
- Place chicken in the greased air fryer. I was able to fit two pieces of chicken in my air fryer at a time.
- Cook at 370 degrees for about 11-13 minutes, or until desired brown-ness. Use tongs to flip it halfway cook time.
- Once finished, cut chicken in half, and place on a hamburger bun. Add desired fixings like pickles and mayonnaise.

Nutrition info

Calories 233 Calories from Fat 117, Fat 11g, Saturated Fat 2g, Cholesterol 94mg, Sodium 75mg, Potassium 833mg, Protein 27g

142.Sheet Pan Shakshuka

Try out this unique egg dish with some toasted bread!

Prep time and cooking time: 25 minutes | Serves: 4

Ingredients to Use:

4 large eggs

1 large Anaheim chili, chopped

2 tbsp. vegetable oil

1/2 cup onion, chopped

1 tsp. cumin, ground

2 minced garlic cloves

1/2 cup feta cheese

1/2 tsp. paprika

1 can of tomatoes

Salt & pepper

Step-by-Step Directions to cook it:

1.   Saute the chili and onions in vegetable oil until tender.

2.   Pour in the remaining ingredients except for eggs and cook until thick.

3.   Make 4 pockets to pour in the eggs.

4.   Bake for 10 minutes at 191̲0̲C or 375̲0̲F in the PowerXL Air Fryer Grill.

5.   Top it off with feta.

Nutritional value per serving:

Calories: 219kcal, Carbs: 20g, Protein: 10g, Fat: 11g.

143. Quick and Easy Air Fryer BBQ Chicken Wings

Prep/Cook Time 25 minutes, Servings :4

Ingredients

- 1.75 lb chicken wings (roughly)
- 1 tsp garlic powder
- 1 tsp smoked paprika
- salt and pepper
- 1 tsp olive oil (plus oil spray)
- 2 tbsp barbecue sauce (or more)

Instructions

- In a large mixing bowl combine chicken wings with garlic powder, smoked paprika, oil, salt, and pepper. Mix well.
- Preheat the Air Fryer to 360F.
- Spread chicken wings on the wire mesh evenly in a single layer. Then cook the wings for about 12 min.
- Flip the wings or just toss the wings for a few seconds and cook further for 5 min.
- Take out out the wings in a mixing bowl. Add barbecue sauce and mix well.
- Cook the coated chicken wings for an additional 2 min.
- Serve warm.

Notes

- Spray some oil using an oil spray on the wire basket before placing the chicken wings. Or lightly brush the oil on the wire mesh. It will help prevent sticking the wings to the basket.
- You can add more barbecue sauce than mentioned in the list as per your likings.

Nutrition Info

Calories: 330kcal, carbohydrates; 26 g protein; 107 mg cholesterol; 311 mg sodium.

144. Air Fryer Whole Chicken

Prep/Cook Time: 1 hr, Servings: people

Ingredients

For a 5 qt. Air fryer:

- 3 lbs whole chicken
- 1.5 tsp coarse salt
- ¼ tsp each black pepper, sweet paprika
- ½ tsp each garlic, onion powder,
- ½ tsp each dry rosemary, dry thyme (or 1 tsp Italian seasoning)

For a 6 qt. Air fryer:

- 4 lbs whole chicken
- 2 tsp coarse salt
- 1/4 tsp each black pepper, sweet paprika
- ½ tsp each garlic, onion powder,
- ½ tsp each dry rosemary, dry thyme (or 1 tsp Italian seasoning)

Instructions

- Remove the giblets inside the whole chicken cavity. Pat dry with a clean paper towel.
- Combine dry spice seasonings from salt to thyme in a bowl.
- Use your fingers to gently separate the skin from the meat to create small pockets. Be careful not to tear the skin. Stuff the dry spice mixture under the skin and use your hands to gently spread the spices as even as you can. Make sure to season the outer interior and the back of the bird.
- Place the whole chicken breast side down in the air fryer. Roast at 360F for 30 minutes.
- Flip the chicken (now breast side up and roast at the same temperature for 20 minutes (3 lbs. chicken) or 25 minutes (4 lbs. chicken).
- Test the internal temperature with a meat thermometer. It should reach at least 165F at the thickest part without touching the bones. If not, send it back and roast for 5 additional minutes then test the temperature again.
- Allow the chicken to rest for 10 minutes before carving. The bottom of the air fryer basket will catch all the chicken juice. Serve the juice on the side if you like.

Nutrition Info

Calories: 356kcal, Carbohydrates: 1g, Protein: 31g, Fat: 25g, Saturated Fat: 7g, Cholesterol: 122mg, Sodium: 115mg, Potassium: 326mg, Fiber: 1g, Sugar: 1g, Calcium: 18mg, Iron: 1.6mg

145. Air Fryer Chicken Nuggets

Prep/Cook Time: 22 minutes, Servings: 4 servings

Ingredients

- 1/4 cup whole wheat flour
- 1/4 teaspoon salt, or to taste
- 1/4 teaspoon black pepper

- 1 large egg
- 2/3 cup whole wheat panko bread crumbs
- 1/3 cup grated Parmesan cheese
- 2 teaspoons dried parsley flakes
- 1 pound boneless, skinless chicken breasts, cut into 1-inch cubes
- Olive oil spray
- Optional dipping sauce: marinara or pizza sauce, barbecue sauce, or ranch dressing

Instructions

- Preheat air fryer at 400ºF for 8-10 minutes.
- Set out three small shallow bowls. In the first bowl, place flour, salt, and pepper; mix lightly. In the second bowl, add egg and beat lightly.
- In the third bowl, combine Panko, parmesan cheese,and parsley flakes.
- One at a time, coat chicken pieces in the flour mixture, then dip into the beaten egg, and finally coat with the Panko mixture, pressing lightly to help the coating adhere.
- Place chicken nuggets in basket of air fryer, in a single layer. Spray the nuggets with olive oil spray (this helps them get golden brown and crispy). You will not be able to cook them all at once. Cook each batch of chicken nuggets for 7 minutes, or until internal temperature reaches 165ºF. Do not overcook.

Nutrition Info

Calories: 399, Total Fat: 8g, Saturated Fat: 3g, Cholesterol: 150mg, Sodium: 434mg, Carbohydrates: 34g, Fiber: 5g, Sugar: 1g, Protein: 46g

146.Air Fryer Chicken Teriyaki Bowls

Prep/Cook Time: 50 minutes, Servings: 6

Ingredients

- 6 Boneless, Skinless Chicken Thighs
- 1/4 Cup Cornstarch or Potato Starch
- 1/2 Cup Gluten-Free or Regular Soy Sauce
- 1/4 Cup Water
- 2 Tbsp Rice Wine Vinegar
- 2 Tbsp Brown Sugar
- 1/4 Cup Granulated Sugar
- 1 Clove Garlic, Crushed
- 1 Tsp Ground Ginger
- 1/2 Tbsp Cornstarch
- 3 Cups Cooked White Rice
- 2 Cups Cooked Green Beans
- 2 Green Onions, Diced

Instructions

- Cut the chicken into cubed chunks, then toss in a bowl with Cornstarch or Potato Starch. Use enough to coat the chicken evenly.
- Place in the Air Fryer and cook according to your Air Fryer Manual for chicken. (Note - I cooked ours on 390* for 10-15 minutes on each side.)
- While the chicken is cooking, in a small saucepan, combine the soy sauce, water, rice wine vinegar, brown sugar, regular sugar, garlic, and ginger. Whisk this well until it's nicely combined.
- Bring this to a low boil, then whisk in the cornstarch until the sauce is thickened. (Note - if it isn't as thick as you prefer, add another 1/2 Tablespoon.)
- Remove from heat for about 5 minutes and let it thicken up.
- Set aside.
- Once the chicken is cooked up to an internal temperature of at least 165 degrees, mix it into the sauce and warm up. This can be done in a small skillet or the saucepan, simply coat the chicken with the sauce.
- Serve the chicken over the cooked rice with green beans.
- Garnish with green onion.

Nutrition Info

Calories: 404 Total Fat: 9g Saturated Fat: 3g, Sugar: 14g, Protein: 34g

147.Air Fryer BBQ Drumsticks

Prep/Cook Time 30 minutes, Servings: 5 servings

Ingredients

- 5-6 chicken drumsticks
- 1/8 cup extra virgin olive oil
- 1/2 teaspoon garlic powder
- 1/4 teaspoon paprika
- 1/4 teaspoon onion powder
- 1/4 teaspoon salt
- 1/8 teaspoon pepper
- 1/2 cup BBQ sauce (I prefer Sweet Baby Ray's)

Optional

- pinch of cayenne pepper to add spice

Instructions

- Preheat your air fryer to 400 degrees.
- Pat drychicken drumsticks.
- Mix together the olive oil, garlic powder, paprika, onion powder, salt and pepper, and cayenne pepper (if using).
- Coat the chicken drumsticks with oil mixture and massage into the drumsticks for a few minutes to help keep the flavor in.
- Add chicken drumsticks to the air fryer in one single layer and cook for 15 minutes.
- Flip chicken and cook for another 5 minutes.
- Baste chicken with BBQ sauce, flip, then baste other side of chicken with BBQ sauce.
- Cook until chicken has an internal temperature of 165 degrees, about 3-5 more minutes.
- Remove from the air fryer, baste additional BBQ sauce if desired and enjoy!

Nutrition Info

Calories: 297, Total Fat: 15g, Saturated Fat: 3g, Trans Unsaturated Fat: 10g, Cholesterol: 139mg, Sodium: 503mg, Carbohydrates: 12g, Sugar: 9g, Protein: 27g

148.Chicken Curry Salad

You can even take the healthy route with a PowerXL Air Fryer Grill. Go on and make a chicken salad.

Prep time and cooking time: 55 minutes | Serves: 4

Ingredients to Use:

3 chicken breasts cut into cubes

1 tbsp. Dijon mustard

1/2 cup of mayo

Chopped celery

A cup of red grapes, cut into halves

1 tbsp. sour cream

Salt and pepper for seasoning

2 tbsp. cilantro, chopped

1-1/2 tbsp. of spice mix

Step-by-Step Directions to cook it:

1. *Cook boneless chicken for half an hour at 149$\underline{0}$C or 300$\underline{0}$F in the PowerXL Air Fryer Grill.*
2. *Combine the remaining ingredients.*
3. *Add the cooked chicken and grapes to the mixture. Mix them well.*
4. *Put a plastic wrap on the bowl and refrigerate overnight before serving.*

Nutritional value per serving:

Calories: 325kcal, Carbs: 13g, Protein: 37g, Fat: 14g.

CHAPTER 6 VEGAN AND VEGETARIAN

149.Onion Rings

Preparation Time: 10 minutes
Cooking Time: 10 minutes
Servings: 3
Ingredients:
- 2 white onions, sliced into rings
- 1 cup flour
- 2 eggs, beaten
- 1 cup breadcrumbs

Method:
1. Cover the onion rings with flour.
2. Dip in the egg.
3. Dredge with breadcrumbs.
4. Add to the air fryer.
5. Set it to air fry.
6. Cook at 400 degrees F for 10 minutes.

Serving Suggestions: *Serve with tartar sauce.*
Preparation & Cooking Tips: *Make ahead of time and freeze. Air fry when ready to serve.*

150.Cauliflower Bites

Preparation Time: 15 minutes
Cooking Time: 10 minutes
Servings: 6
Ingredients:
Cauliflower bites
- 4 cups cauliflower rice
- 1 egg, beaten
- 1 cup Parmesan cheese, grated
- 1 cup cheddar, shredded
- 2 tablespoons chives, chopped
- ¼ cup breadcrumbs
- Salt and pepper to taste

Sauce
- ½ cup ketchup
- 2 tablespoons hot sauce

Method:
1. Combine cauliflower bites ingredients in a bowl.
2. Mix well.
3. Form balls from the mixture.
4. Choose air fry setting.
5. Add cauliflower bites to the air fryer.
6. Cook at 375 degrees F for 10 minutes.
7. Mix ketchup and hot sauce.
8. Serve cauliflower bites with dip.

Serving Suggestions: *Garnish with chopped parsley.*
Preparation & Cooking Tips: *You can make your own cauliflower rice by pulsing cauliflower florets in a food processor.*

151.Balsamic Asparagus Spears

Prep time: 15 minutes | Cook time: 10 minutes | Serves 4

4 tablespoons olive oil, plus more for greasing
4 tablespoons balsamic vinegar
1½ pounds (680 g) asparagus spears, trimmed
Salt and freshly ground black pepper, to taste

1. Grease the air fry basket with olive oil.
2. In a shallow bowl, stir together the 4 tablespoons of olive oil and balsamic vinegar to make a marinade.
3. Put the asparagus spears in the bowl so they are thoroughly covered by the marinade and allow to marinate for 5 minutes.
4. Put the asparagus in the greased basket in a single layer and season with salt and pepper.
5. Place the air fry basket on the air fry position.
6. Select Air Fry, set temperature to 350ºF (180ºC), and set time to 10 minutes. Flip the asparagus halfway through the cooking time.
7. When done, the asparagus should be tender and lightly browned. Cool for 5 minutes before serving.

152.Baked Potatoes

Preparation Time: 20 minutes
Cooking Time: 45 minutes
Servings: 6
Ingredients:
- 6 potatoes
- 1 tablespoon olive oil
- Salt to taste
- 1 cup butter
- ½ cup milk
- ½ cup sour cream
- 1 ½ cup cheddar, shredded and divided

Method:

1. Poke the potatoes using a fork.
2. Add to the air fryer.
3. Set it to bake.
4. Cook at 400 degrees F for 40 minutes.
5. Take out of the oven.
6. Slice the potato in half
7. Scoop out the potato flesh.
8. Mix potato flesh with the remaining ingredients.
9. Put the mixture back to the potato shells.
10. Bake in the air fryer for 5 minutes.

Serving Suggestions: *Garnish with chopped green onions.*

Preparation & Cooking Tips: *Use large Russet potatoes.*

153.Cheesy Egg Rolls

Preparation Time: 15 minutes
Cooking Time: 12 minutes
Servings: 12

Ingredients:
- 12 spring roll wrappers
- 12 slices provolone cheese
- 3 eggs, cooked and sliced
- 1 carrot, sliced into thin strips
- 1 tablespoon water

Method:
1. Top the wrappers with cheese, eggs and carrot strips.
2. Roll up the wrappers and seal with water.
3. Place inside the air fryer.
4. Set it to air fry.
5. Cook at 390 degrees F for 12 minutes, turning once or twice.

Serving Suggestions: *Serve with ketchup or sweet chili sauce.*

Preparation & Cooking Tips: *You can also use cheddar cheese for this recipe.*

154.Vegetarian Pizza

Preparation Time: 15 minutes
Cooking Time: 10 minutes
Servings: 1

Ingredients:
- 1 pizza crust
- 1 tablespoon olive oil
- ¼ cup tomato sauce
- 1 cup mushrooms
- ½ cup black olives, sliced
- 1 clove garlic, minced
- ½ teaspoon oregano
- Salt and pepper to taste
- 1 cup mozzarella, shredded

Method:
1. Brush pizza crust with oil.
2. Spread tomato sauce on top.
3. Arrange mushrooms and olives on top.
4. Sprinkle with garlic and oregano.
5. Season with salt and pepper.
6. Top with mozzarella cheese.
7. Place inside the air fryer.
8. Set it to bake.
9. Cook at 400 degrees F for 10 minutes.

Serving Suggestions: *Garnish with fresh basil leaves.*

Preparation & Cooking Tips: *Use 8-inch diameter pizza crust.*

155.Brussels Sprout Chips

Preparation Time: 10 minutes
Cooking Time: 15 minutes
Servings: 2

Ingredients:
- 2 cups Brussels sprouts, sliced thinly
- 1 tablespoon olive oil
- 1 teaspoon garlic powder
- Salt and pepper to taste
- 2 tablespoons Parmesan cheese, grated

Method:
1. Toss the Brussels sprouts in oil.
2. Sprinkle with garlic powder, salt, pepper and Parmesan cheese.
3. Choose bake function.
4. Add the Brussels sprouts in the air fryer.
5. Cook at 350 degrees F for 8 minutes.
6. Flip and cook for 7 more minutes.

Serving Suggestions: *Serve with Caesar dressing for dipping.*

Preparation & Cooking Tips: *You can also use this recipe for other vegetables like cauliflower or broccoli.*

156.Golden Eggplant Slices with Parsley

Prep time: 5 minutes | Cook time: 12 minutes | Serves 4

1 cup flour

4 eggs

Salt, to taste

2 cups bread crumbs

1 teaspoon Italian seasoning

2 eggplants, sliced

2 garlic cloves, sliced

2 tablespoons chopped parsley

Cooking spray

1. Spritz the air fry basket with cooking spray. Set aside.

2. On a plate, place the flour. In a shallow bowl, whisk the eggs with salt. In another shallow bowl, combine the bread crumbs and Italian seasoning.

3. Dredge the eggplant slices, one at a time, in the flour, then in the whisked eggs, finally in the bread crumb mixture to coat well.

4. Lay the coated eggplant slices in the air fry basket.

5. Place the basket on the air fry position.

6. Select Air Fry, set temperature to 390ºF (199ºC), and set time to 12 minutes. Flip the eggplant slices halfway through the cooking time.

7. When cooking is complete, the eggplant slices should be golden brown and crispy. Transfer the eggplant slices to a plate and sprinkle the parsley and garlic on top before serving.

157.Toasted-Baked Tofu cubes

Here's simple and easy toasted tofu you can indulge in a matter of minutes.

Prep Time and Cooking Time: 30 minutes | Serves: 2

Ingredients To Use:

1/2 block of tofu, cubed

1 tbsp. olive oil

1 tbsp. nutritional yeast

1 tbsp. flour

1/4 tsp. black pepper

1 tsp. sea salt

1/2 tsp. garlic powder

Step-by-Step Directions to cook it:

1. **Combine all the ingredients with tofu**

2. **Preheat the PowerXL Air Fryer Grill at 230ºC or 400ºF.**

3. Bake tofu on a lined baking tray for 15-30 minutes, turn it around every 10 minutes.

Nutritional value per serving:

Calories: 100kcal, Carbs: 5g, Protein: 8g, Fat 6g.

158.Veggie Rolls

Preparation Time: 20 minutes

Cooking Time: 20 minutes

Servings: 5

Ingredients:

- 1 tablespoon olive oil
- 1 clove garlic, minced
- 1 teaspoon ginger, minced
- 3 scallions, chopped
- ½ lb. mushrooms, chopped
- 2 cups cabbage, chopped
- 8 oz. water chestnuts, diced
- Salt and pepper to taste
- 6 spring roll wrappers
- 1 tablespoon water

Method:

1. Add oil to a pan over medium heat.

2. Cook the garlic, ginger, scallions and mushrooms for 2 minutes.

3. Stir in the remaining vegetables.

4. Season with salt and pepper.

5. Cook for 3 minutes, stirring.

6. Transfer to a strainer.

7. Add vegetables on top of the wrappers.

8. Roll up the wrappers.

9. Seal the edges with water.

10. Place the rolls inside the air fryer.

11. Choose air fry setting.

12. Cook at 360 degrees F for 15 minutes.

Serving Suggestions: *Serve with vinegar dipping sauce.*

Preparation & Cooking Tips: Cook in batches.

159.Toasted Vegetables with Rice and Eggs

Prep time: 5 minutes | Cook time: 12 minutes | Serves 4

2 teaspoons melted butter

1 cup chopped mushrooms

1 cup cooked rice

1 cup peas

1 carrot, chopped

1 red onion, chopped

1 garlic clove, minced

Salt and black pepper, to taste

2 hard-boiled eggs, grated

1 tablespoon soy sauce

1.   Coat a baking dish with melted butter.

2.   Stir together the mushrooms, carrot, peas, garlic, onion, cooked rice, salt, and pepper in a large bowl until well mixed. Pour the mixture into the prepared baking dish.

3.   Place the baking dish on the toast position.

4.   Select Toast, set temperature to 380ºF (193ºC), and set time to 12 minutes.

5.   When cooking is complete, remove from the air fryer grill. Divide the mixture among four plates. Serve warm with a sprinkle of grated eggs and a drizzle of soy sauce.

160.Lemony Brussels Sprouts

Prep time: 15 minutes | Cook time: 20 minutes | Serves 4

1 pound (454 g) Brussels sprouts, trimmed and halved

1 tablespoon extra-virgin olive oil

Sea Salt and freshly ground black pepper, to taste

½ cup sun-dried tomatoes, chopped

2 tablespoons freshly squeezed lemon juice

1 teaspoon lemon zest

1.   Line a large baking sheet with aluminum foil.

2.   Toss the Brussels sprouts with the olive oil in a large bowl. Sprinkle with salt and black pepper.

3.   Spread the Brussels sprouts in a single layer on the baking sheet.

4.   Place the baking sheet on the toast position.

5.   Select Toast, set temperature to 400ºF (205ºC), and set time to 20 minutes.

6.   When done, the Brussels sprouts should be caramelized. Remove from the air fryer grill to a serving bowl, along with the tomatoes, lemon juice, and lemon zest. Toss to combine. Serve immediately.

161.Zucchini Lasagna

Preparation Time: 15 minutes

Cooking Time: 15 minutes

Servings: 4

Ingredients:

- 1 zucchini, sliced thinly lengthwise and divided
- ½ cup marinara sauce, divided
- ¼ cup ricotta, divided
- 1 cup fresh basil leaves, chopped and divided
- ¼ cup spinach leaves, chopped and divided

Method:

1.   Layer half of the zucchini slices in a small loaf pan.

2.   Spread with half of marinara sauce and ricotta.

3.   Top with half of spinach and basil.

4.   Repeat layers with the remaining ingredients.

5.   Cover the pan with foil.

6.   Place inside the air fryer.

7.   Set it to bake.

8.   Cook at 400 degrees F for 10 minutes.

9.   Remove foil and cook for another 5 minutes.

Serving Suggestions: *Garnish with fresh basil.*

Preparation & Cooking Tips: *Make this ahead of time by freezing and baking when ready to serve.*

162.Eggplant Pizza

A delicious gluten-free pizza to curb your cravings.

Prep Time and Cooking Time: 45 minutes | Serves: 2

Ingredients To Use:

Eggplant (sliced 1/4 -inch)

Gluten-free pizza dough

1 cup pizza sauce

Fresh rosemary and basil

Cheese

Garlic cloves, chopped

Red pepper, salt, and pepper

Olive oil

Step-by-Step Directions to cook it:

1.   **Rub eggplant slices with olive oil and rosemary, salt and pepper, and bake for 25 mins at 218̲0̲C or 425̲0̲F in the PowerXL Air Fryer Grill**

2.   **Roll the dough round and spread the remaining ingredients on top.**

3.   **Preheat the PowerXL Air Fryer Grill at 230̲0̲C or 450̲0̲F at pizza-setting and bake the pizza for 10 minutes.**

Nutritional value per serving:

Calories: 260kcal, Carbs: 24g, Protein: 9g, Fat 14g.

163. Cheesy Stuffed Mushrooms with Veggies

Prep time: 5 minutes | Cook time: 8 minutes | Serves 4

4 portobello mushrooms, stem removed
1 tablespoon olive oil
1 tomato, diced
½ green bell pepper, diced
½ small red onion, diced
½ teaspoon garlic powder
Salt and black pepper, to taste
½ cup grated Mozzarella cheese

1.   Using a spoon to scoop out the gills of the mushrooms and discard them. Brush the mushrooms with the olive oil.
2.   In a mixing bowl, stir together the remaining ingredients except the Mozzarella cheese. Using a spoon to stuff each mushroom with the filling and scatter the Mozzarella cheese on top.
3.   Arrange the mushrooms in the air fry basket.
4.   Place the basket on the toast position.
5.   Select Toast, set temperature to 330ºF (166ºC) and set time to 8 minutes.
6.   When cooking is complete, the cheese should be melted.
7.   Serve warm.

164. Toasted Mushrooms, Pepper and Squash

Prep time: 10 minutes | Cook time: 16 minutes | Serves 4

1 (8-ounce / 227-g) package sliced mushrooms
1 yellow summer squash, sliced
1 red bell pepper, sliced
3 cloves garlic, sliced
1 tablespoon olive oil
½ teaspoon dried basil
½ teaspoon dried thyme
½ teaspoon dried tarragon

1.   Toss the mushrooms, bell pepper, and squash with the garlic and olive oil in a large bowl until well coated. Mix in the basil, thyme, and tarragon and toss again.
2.   Spread the vegetables evenly in the air fry basket.
3.   Place the basket on the toast position.
4.   Select Toast, set temperature to 350ºF (180ºC), and set time to 16 minutes.
5.   When cooking is complete, the vegetables should be fork-tender. Remove the basket from the air fryer grill. Cool for 5 minutes before serving.

165. Fast Lemony Wax Beans

Prep time: 5 minutes | Cook time: 12 minutes | Serves 4

2 pounds (907 g) wax beans
2 tablespoons extra-virgin olive oil
Salt and freshly ground black pepper, to taste
Juice of ½ lemon, for serving

1.   Line a baking sheet with aluminum foil.
2.   Toss the wax beans with the olive oil in a large bowl. Lightly season with pepper and salt.
3.   Spread out the wax beans on the sheet pan.
4.   Place the baking sheet on the toast position.
5.   Select Toast, set temperature to 400ºF (205ºC), and set time to 12 minutes.
6.   When done, the beans will be caramelized and tender. Remove from the air fryer grill to a plate and serve sprinkled with the lemon juice.

166. Sriracha Roasted Potatoes

Try some spicy roasted potatoes to make your day.
Prep Time and Cooking Time: 40 minutes | Servings: 3

Ingredients To Use:
3 potatoes, diced
2-3 tsp. sriracha
1/4 garlic powder
Salt & pepper
Olive oil
Chopped fresh parsley

Step-by-Step Directions to cook it:
1.   **Combine the potatoes with the remaining ingredients.**
2.   **Preheat the PowerXL Air Fryer Grill at 230ᴑC or 450ᴑF.**
3.   **Line the pan with olive oil and spread the coated potatoes. Sprinkle parsley.**
4.   **Bake for 30 minutes.**

Nutritional value per serving:
Calories 147kcal, Carbs: 24.4, Protein: 3g, Fat 4.7g.

CHAPTER 7 VEGETABLE SIDES

167. Garlicky-Balsamic Asparagus

Prep time: 5 minutes | Cook time: 10 minutes | Serves 4

1 pound (454 g) asparagus, woody ends trimmed
2 tablespoons olive oil
1 tablespoon balsamic vinegar
2 teaspoons minced garlic
Salt and freshly ground black pepper, to taste

1. In a large shallow bowl, toss the asparagus with the garlic, balsamic vinegar, olive oil, salt, and pepper until thoroughly coated. Put the asparagus in the air fry basket.
2. Place the basket on the toast position.
3. Select Toast, set temperature to 400ºF (205ºC), and set time to 10 minutes. Flip the asparagus with tongs halfway through the cooking time.
4. When cooking is complete, the asparagus should be crispy. Remove the basket from the air fryer grill and serve warm.

168. Cheesy Buttered Broccoli

Prep time: 5 minutes | Cook time: 4 minutes | Serves 4

1 pound (454 g) broccoli florets
1 medium shallot, minced
2 tablespoons olive oil
2 tablespoons unsalted butter, melted
2 teaspoons minced garlic
¼ cup grated Parmesan cheese

1. Combine the broccoli florets with the butter, garlic, shallot, olive oil, and Parmesan cheese in a medium bowl and toss until the broccoli florets are thoroughly coated.
2. Place the broccoli florets in the air fry basket in a single layer.
3. Place the basket on the toast position.
4. Select Toast, set temperature to 360ºF (182ºC), and set time to 4 minutes.
5. When cooking is complete, the broccoli florets should be crisp-tender. Remove from the air fryer grill and serve warm.

169. Broccoli with Hot Sauce

Prep time: 5 minutes | Cook time: 14 minutes | Serves 6

Broccoli:
1 medium-sized head broccoli, cut into florets
1½ tablespoons olive oil
1 teaspoon shallot powder
1 teaspoon porcini powder
½ teaspoon freshly grated lemon zest
½ teaspoon hot paprika
½ teaspoon granulated garlic
$1/_3$ teaspoon fine sea salt
$1/_3$ teaspoon celery seeds

Hot Sauce:
½ cup tomato sauce
1 tablespoon balsamic vinegar
½ teaspoon ground allspice

1. In a mixing bowl, combine all the ingredients for the broccoli and toss to coat. Transfer the broccoli to the air fry basket.
2. Place the basket on the air fry position.
3. Select Air Fry, set temperature to 360ºF (182ºC), and set time to 14 minutes.
4. Meanwhile, make the hot sauce by whisking together the balsamic vinegar, tomato sauce, and allspice in a small bowl.
5. When cooking is complete, remove the broccoli from the air fryer grill and serve with the hot sauce.

170. Crispy Brussels Sprouts with Sage

Prep time: 5 minutes | Cook time: 15 minutes | Serves 4

1 pound (454 g) Brussels sprouts, halved
1 cup bread crumbs
2 tablespoons grated Grana Padano cheese
1 tablespoon paprika
2 tablespoons canola oil
1 tablespoon chopped sage

1. Line the air fry basket with parchment paper. Set aside.
2. In a small bowl, thoroughly mix the cheese, bread crumbs, and paprika. In a large bowl, place the Brussels sprouts and drizzle the canola oil over the top. Sprinkle with the bread crumb mixture and toss to coat.
3. Transfer the Brussels sprouts to the prepared basket.
4. Place the basket on the toast position.
5. Select Toast, set temperature to 400ºF (205ºC), and set time to 15 minutes. Stir the Brussels a few times during cooking.

When cooking is complete, the Brussels sprouts should be lightly browned and crisp. Transfer the Brussels sprouts to a plate and sprinkle the sage on top before serving

CHAPTER 8 APPETIZERS AND SNACKS

171.Cheesy Pepperoni Pizza Bites

Prep time: 5 minutes | Cook time: 12 minutes | Serves 8

1 cup finely shredded Mozzarella cheese

½ cup chopped pepperoni

¼ cup Marinara sauce

1 (8-ounce / 227-g) can crescent roll dough

All-purpose flour, for dusting

1.   In a small bowl, stir together the cheese, pepperoni, and Marinara sauce.

2.   Lay the dough on a lightly floured work surface. Separate it into 4 rectangles. Firmly pinch the perforations together and pat the dough pieces flat.

3.   Divide the cheese mixture evenly between the rectangles and spread it out over the dough, leaving a ¼-inch border. Roll a rectangle up tightly, starting with the short end. Pinch the edge down to seal the roll. Repeat with the remaining rolls.

4.   Slice the rolls into 4 or 5 even slices. Place the slices on the sheet pan, leaving a few inches between each slice.

5.   Place the pan on the toast position.

6.   Select Toast, set temperature to 350ºF (180ºC) and set time to 12 minutes.

7.   After 6 minutes, rotate the pan and continue cooking.

8.   When cooking is complete, the rolls will be golden brown with crisp edges. Remove the pan from the air fryer grill. Serve hot.

172.Crispy Kale Chips

Prep time: 15 minutes | Cook time: 8 minutes | Serves 5

8 cups deribbed kale leaves, torn into 2-inch pieces

1½ tablespoons olive oil

¾ teaspoon chili powder

¼ teaspoon garlic powder

½ teaspoon paprika

2 teaspoons sesame seeds

1.   In a large bowl, toss the kale with the olive oil, garlic powder, chili powder, sesame seeds, and paprika until well coated.

2.   Transfer the kale to the air fry basket.

3.   Place the basket on the air fry position.

4.   Select Air Fry, set temperature to 350ºF (180ºC), and set time to 8 minutes. Flip the kale twice during cooking.

5.   When cooking is complete, the kale should be crispy. Remove from the air fryer grill and serve warm.

173.Golden Cornmeal Batter Ball

Prep time: 45 minutes | Cook time: 10 minutes | Serves 12

1 cup self-rising yellow cornmeal

½ cup all-purpose flour

1 teaspoon sugar

1 teaspoon salt

1 teaspoon freshly ground black pepper

1 large egg

$^1/_3$ cup canned creamed corn

1 cup minced onion

2 teaspoons minced jalapeño pepper

2 tablespoons olive oil, divided

1.   Thoroughly combine the flour, cornmeal, salt, sugar, and pepper in a large bowl.

2.   Whisk together the egg and corn in a small bowl. Pour the egg mixture into the bowl of cornmeal mixture and stir to combine. Stir in the jalapeño and minced onion. Cover the bowl with plastic wrap and place in the refrigerator for 30 minutes.

3.   Line the air fry basket with parchment paper and lightly brush it with 1 tablespoon of olive oil.

4.   Scoop out the cornmeal mixture and form into 24 balls, about 1 inch.

5.   Arrange the balls on the parchment, leaving space between each ball.

6.   Place the basket on the air fry position.

7.   Select Air Fry, set temperature to 375ºF (190ºC), and set time to 10 minutes.

8.   After 5 minutes, remove the basket from the air fryer grill. Flip the balls and brush them with the remaining 1 tablespoon of olive oil. Return to the air fryer grill and continue cooking for 5 minutes until golden brown.

9.   When cooking is complete, remove the balls (hush puppies) from the air fryer grill and serve on a plate.

174.Bacon Onion Rings

Preparation Time: 15 minutes
Cooking Time: 10 minutes
Servings: 4
Ingredients:
- 2 white onions, sliced into rings
- 1 tablespoon hot sauce
- 10 bacon slices

Method:
1.   Coat onion rings with hot sauce.
2.   Wrap each onion ring with bacon.
3.   Add to the air fryer.
4.   Set it to air fry.
5.   Cook at 370 degrees F for 5 minutes per side.

Serving Suggestions: ***Serve with mayo and ketchup.***
Preparation & Cooking Tips: ***You can also brush onion rings with olive oil instead of hot sauce.***

175..Cinnamon Apple Wedges with Yogurt

Prep time: 10 minutes | Cook time: 12 minutes | Serves 4
2 medium apples, cored and sliced into ¼-inch wedges
1 teaspoon canola oil
2 teaspoons peeled and grated fresh ginger
½ teaspoon ground cinnamon
½ cup low-fat Greek vanilla yogurt, for serving
1.   In a large bowl, toss the apple wedges with the cinnamon, ginger, and canola oil until evenly coated. Put the apple wedges in the air fry basket.
2.   Place the basket on the air fry position.
3.   Select Air Fry, set temperature to 360ºF (182ºC), and set time to 12 minutes.
4.   When cooking is complete, the apple wedges should be crisp-tender. Remove the apple wedges from the air fryer grill and serve drizzled with the yogurt.

176.Hot Corn Tortilla Chips

Prep time: 5 minutes | Cook time: 5 minutes | Serves 4
½ teaspoon ground cumin

½ teaspoon paprika
½ teaspoon chili powder
½ teaspoon salt
Pinch cayenne pepper
8 (6-inch) corn tortillas, each cut into 6 wedges
Cooking spray
1.   Lightly spritz the air fry basket with cooking spray.
2.   Stir together the paprika, chili powder, cumin, salt, and pepper in a small bowl.
3.   Place the tortilla wedges in the air fry basket in a single layer. Lightly mist them with cooking spray. Sprinkle the seasoning mixture on top of the tortilla wedges.
4.   Place the basket on the air fry position.
5.   Select Air Fry, set temperature to 375ºF (190ºC), and set time to 5 minutes. Stir the tortilla wedges halfway through the cooking time.
6.   When cooking is complete, the chips should be lightly browned and crunchy. Remove the basket from the air fryer grill. Let the tortilla chips cool for 5 minutes and serve.

177.Cheesy Jalapeño Peppers

Prep time: 10 minutes | Cook time: 15 minutes | Serves 8
6 ounces (170 g) cream cheese, at room temperature
4 ounces (113 g) shredded Cheddar cheese
1 teaspoon chili powder
12 large jalapeño peppers, deseeded and sliced in half lengthwise
2 slices cooked bacon, chopped
¼ cup panko bread crumbs
1 tablespoon butter, melted
1.   In a medium bowl, whisk together the Cheddar cheese, cream cheese, and chili powder. Spoon the cheese mixture into the jalapeño halves and arrange them on the sheet pan.
2.   In a small bowl, stir together the bacon, butter and bread crumbs. Sprinkle the mixture over the jalapeño halves.
3.   Place the pan on the toast position.
4.   Select Toast, set temperature to 375ºF (190ºC) and set time to 15 minutes.
5.   After 7 or 8 minutes, rotate the pan and continue cooking until the peppers are softened, the filling is bubbling and the bread crumbs are browned.

6.   When cooking is complete, remove the pan from the air fryer grill. Let the poppers cool for 5 minutes before serving.

Simple Sweet Cinnamon Peaches

Prep time: 5 minutes | Cook time: 10 minutes | Serves 4

2 tablespoons sugar
¼ teaspoon ground cinnamon
4 peaches, cut into wedges
Cooking spray

1.   Spritz the air fry basket with cooking spray.
2.   In a large bowl, stir together the sugar and cinnamon. Add the peaches to the bowl and toss to coat evenly.
3.   Spread the coated peaches in a single layer in the air fry basket.
4.   Place the basket on the air fry position.
5.   Select Air Fry, set temperature to 350ºF (180ºC) and set time to 10 minutes.
6.   After 5 minutes, remove the basket from the air fryer grill. Use tongs to turn the peaches skin side down. Lightly mist them with cooking spray. Return the basket to the air fryer grill to continue cooking.
7.   When cooking is complete, the peaches will be lightly browned and caramelized. Remove the basket from the air fryer grill and let rest for 5 minutes before serving.

178.Crunchy Cod Fingers

Prep time: 5 minutes | Cook time: 12 minutes | Serves 4

2 eggs
2 tablespoons milk
2 cups flour
1 cup cornmeal
1 teaspoon seafood seasoning
Salt and black pepper, to taste
1 cup bread crumbs
1 pound (454 g) cod fillets, cut into 1-inch strips

1.   Beat the eggs with the milk in a shallow bowl. In another shallow bowl, combine the flour, salt, seafood seasoning, cornmeal, and pepper. On a plate, place the bread crumbs.
2.   Dredge the cod strips, one at a time, in the flour mixture, then in the egg mixture, finally roll in the bread crumb to coat evenly.

3.   Transfer the cod strips to the air fry basket.
4.   Place the basket on the air fry position.
5.   Select Air Fry, set temperature to 400ºF (205ºC), and set time to 12 minutes.
6.   When cooking is complete, the cod strips should be crispy. Remove from the air fryer grill to a paper towel-lined plate and serve warm.

179.Crispy Cheesy Mixed Snack

Prep time: 5 minutes | Cook time: 6 minutes | Makes 6 cups

2 cups oyster crackers
2 cups Chex rice
1 cup sesame sticks
$^2/_3$ cup finely grated Parmesan cheese
8 tablespoons unsalted butter, melted
1½ teaspoons granulated garlic
½ teaspoon kosher salt

1.   Toss together all the ingredients in a large bowl until well coated. Spread the mixture on the sheet pan in an even layer.
2.   Place the pan on the toast position.
3.   Select Toast, set temperature to 350ºF (180ºC) and set time to 6 minutes.
4.   After 3 minutes, remove the pan and stir the mixture. Return the pan to the air fryer grill and continue cooking.
5.   When cooking is complete, the mixture should be lightly browned and fragrant. Let cool before serving.

180..Crispy Cheesy Zucchini Tots

Prep time: 15 minutes | Cook time: 6 minutes | Serves 8

2 medium zucchini (about 12 ounces / 340 g), shredded
1 large egg, whisked
½ cup grated pecorino romano cheese
½ cup panko bread crumbs
¼ teaspoon black pepper
1 clove garlic, minced
Cooking spray

1.   Using your hands, squeeze out as much liquid from the zucchini as possible. In a large bowl, mix the zucchini with the remaining ingredients except the oil until well incorporated.

2. Make the zucchini tots: Use a spoon or cookie scoop to place tablespoonfuls of the zucchini mixture onto a lightly floured cutting board and form into 1-inch logs.

3. Spritz the air fry basket with cooking spray. Place the zucchini tots in the pan.

4. Place the basket on the air fry position.

5. Select Air Fry, set temperature to 375ºF (190ºC), and set time to 6 minutes.

6. When cooking is complete, the tots should be golden brown. Remove from the air fryer grill to a serving plate and serve warm.

181.Cheesy BBQ Chicken Pizza

Prep time: 5 minutes | Cook time: 8 minutes | Serves 1

1 piece naan bread
¼ cup Barbecue sauce
¼ cup shredded Monterrey Jack cheese
¼ cup shredded Mozzarella cheese
½ chicken herby sausage , sliced
2 tablespoons red onion, thinly sliced
Chopped cilantro or parsley, for garnish
Cooking spray

1. Spritz the bottom of naan bread with cooking spray, then transfer to the air fry basket.

2. Brush with the Barbecue sauce. Top with the sausage, cheeses, and finish with the red onion.

3. Place the basket on the air fry position.

4. Select Air Fry, set temperature to 400ºF (205ºC), and set time to 8 minutes.

5. When cooking is complete, the cheese should be melted. Remove the basket from the air fryer grill. Garnish with the chopped cilantro or parsley before slicing to serve.

182.Crispy Carrot Chips

Prep time: 15 minutes | Cook time: 10 minutes | Serves 4

4 to 5 medium carrots, trimmed and thinly sliced
1 tablespoon olive oil, plus more for greasing
1 teaspoon seasoned salt

1. Toss the carrot slices with 1 tablespoon of olive oil and salt in a medium bowl until thoroughly coated.

2. Grease the air fry basket with the olive oil. Place the carrot slices in the greased pan.

3. Place the basket on the air fry position.

4. Select Air Fry, set temperature to 390ºF (199ºC), and set time to 10 minutes. Stir the carrot slices halfway through the cooking time.

5. When cooking is complete, the chips should be crisp-tender. Remove the basket from the air fryer grill and allow to cool for 5 minutes before serving.

183.Crispy Apple Chips

Prep time: 10 minutes | Cook time: 10 minutes | Serves 4

4 medium apples (any type will work), cored and thinly sliced
¼ teaspoon nutmeg
¼ teaspoon cinnamon
Cooking spray

1. Place the apple slices in a large bowl and sprinkle the spices on top. Toss to coat.

2. Put the apple slices in the air fry basket in a single layer and spray them with cooking spray.

3. Place the basket on the air fry position.

4. Select Air Fry, set temperature to 360ºF (182ºC), and set time to 10 minutes. Stir the apple slices halfway through.

5. When cooking is complete, the apple chips should be crispy. Transfer the apple chips to a paper towel-lined plate and rest for 5 minutes before serving.

CHAPTER 9 DESSERTS

184.Easy Vanilla Walnuts Tart

Prep time: 5 minutes | Cook time: 13 minutes | Serves 6

1 cup coconut milk
½ cup walnuts, ground
½ cup Swerve
½ cup almond flour
½ stick butter, at room temperature
2 eggs
1 teaspoon vanilla essence
¼ teaspoon ground cardamom
¼ teaspoon ground cloves
Cooking spray

1.   Coat a baking pan with cooking spray.
2.   Combine all the ingredients except the oil in a large bowl and stir until well blended. Spoon the batter mixture into the baking pan.
3.   Place the pan on the bake position.
4.   Select Bake, set temperature to 360ºF (182ºC), and set time to 13 minutes.
5.   When cooking is complete, a toothpick inserted into the center of the tart should come out clean.
6.   Remove from the air fryer grill and place on a wire rack to cool. Serve immediately.

185.Golden Bananaswith Chocolate Sauce

Prep time: 10 minutes | Cook time: 7 minutes | Serves 6

¼ cup cornstarch
¼ cup plain bread crumbs
1 large egg, beaten
3 bananas, halved crosswise
Cooking spray
Chocolate sauce, for serving

1.   Place the bread crumbs, egg, and cornstarch in three separate bowls.
2.   Roll the bananas in the cornstarch, then in the beaten egg, and finally in the bread crumbs to coat well.
3.   Spritz the air fry basket with cooking spray.
4.   Arrange the banana halves in the air fry basket and mist them with cooking spray.
5.   Place the basket on the air fry position.

6.   Select Air Fry, set temperature to 350ºF (180ºC), and set time to 7 minutes.
7.   After about 5 minutes, flip the bananas and continue to air fry for another 2 minutes.
8.   When cooking is complete, remove the bananas from the air fryer grill to a serving plate. Serve with the chocolate sauce drizzled over the top.

186.Honey Apple-Peach Crumble

Prep time: 10 minutes | Cook time: 11 minutes | Serves 4

1 apple, peeled and chopped
2 peaches, peeled, pitted, and chopped
2 tablespoons honey
½ cup quick-cooking oatmeal
$^1/_3$ cup whole-wheat pastry flour
2 tablespoons unsalted butter, at room temperature
3 tablespoons packed brown sugar
½ teaspoon ground cinnamon

1.   Mix together the peaches, apple, and honey in a baking pan until well incorporated.
2.   In a bowl, combine the pastry flour, butter, oatmeal, brown sugar, and cinnamon and stir to mix well. Spread this mixture evenly over the fruit.
3.   Place the pan on the bake position.
4.   Select Bake, set temperature to 380ºF (193ºC), and set time to 11 minutes.
5.   When cooking is complete, the fruit should be bubbling around the edges and the topping should be golden brown.
6.   Remove from the air fryer grill and serve warm.

187.Baked Berries with Coconut Chip

Prep time: 5 minutes | Cook time: 20 minutes | Serves 6

1 tablespoon butter, melted
12 ounces (340 g) mixed berries
$^1/_3$ cup granulated Swerve
1 teaspoon pure vanilla extract
½ teaspoon ground cinnamon
¼ teaspoon ground cloves
¼ teaspoon grated nutmeg
½ cup coconut chips, for garnish

1.   Coat a baking pan with melted butter.

2.   Put the remaining ingredients except the coconut chips in the prepared baking pan.

3.   Place the pan on the bake position.

4.   Select Bake, set temperature to 330ºF (166ºC), and set time to 20 minutes.

5.   When cooking is complete, remove from the air fryer grill. Serve garnished with the coconut chips.

188. Simple Blackberry Chocolate Cake

Prep time: 10 minutes | Cook time: 22 minutes | Serves 8

½ cup butter, at room temperature

2 ounces (57 g) Swerve

4 eggs

1 cup almond flour

1 teaspoon baking soda

$^1/_3$ teaspoon baking powder

½ cup cocoa powder

1 teaspoon orange zest

$^1/_3$ cup fresh blackberries

1.   With an hand mixer or electric mixer, beat the butter and Swerve until creamy.

2.   One at a time, mix in the eggs and beat again until fluffy.

3.   Add the almond flour, cocoa powder, baking powder, baking soda, orange zest and mix well. Add the butter mixture to the almond flour mixture and stir until well blended. Fold in the blackberries.

4.   Scrape the batter into a baking pan.

5.   Place the pan on the bake position.

6.   Select Bake, set temperature to 335ºF (168ºC), and set time to 22 minutes.

7.   When cooking is complete, a toothpick inserted into the center of the cake should come out clean.

8.   Allow the cake cool on a wire rack to room temperature. Serve immediately.

189. Caramelized Fruit Skewers

Prep time: 10 minutes | Cook time: 4 minutes | Serves 4

2 peaches, peeled, pitted, and thickly sliced

3 plums, halved and pitted

3 nectarines, halved and pitted

1 tablespoon honey

½ teaspoon ground cinnamon

¼ teaspoon ground allspice

Pinch cayenne pepper

Special Equipment:

8 metal skewers

1.   Thread, alternating plums, nectarines, and peaches onto the metal skewers that fit into the air fryer grill.

2.   Thoroughly combine the honey, cayenne, cinnamon, and allspice in a small bowl. Brush generously the glaze over the fruit skewers.

3.   Transfer the fruit skewers to the air fry basket.

4.   Place the basket on the air fry position.

5.   Select Air Fry, set temperature to 400ºF (205ºC), and set time to 4 minutes.

6.   When cooking is complete, the fruit should be caramelized.

7.   Remove the fruit skewers from the air fryer grill and let rest for 5 minutes before serving.

190. Vanilla Chocolate Cookies

Prep time: 10 minutes | Cook time: 22 minutes | Makes 30 cookies

$^1/_3$ cup (80g) organic brown sugar

$^1/_3$ cup (80g) organic cane sugar

4 ounces (112g) cashew-based vegan butter

½ cup coconut cream

1 teaspoon vanilla extract

2 tablespoons ground flaxseed

1 teaspoon baking powder

1 teaspoon baking soda

Pinch of salt

2¼ cups (220g) almond flour

½ cup (90g) dairy-free dark chocolate chips

1.   Line a baking sheet with parchment paper.

2.   Mix together the brown sugar, cane sugar, and butter in a medium bowl or the bowl of a stand mixer. Cream together with a mixer.

3.   Fold in the vanilla, coconut cream, flaxseed, baking soda, baking powder, and salt. Stir well.

4.   Add the almond flour, a little at a time, mixing after each addition until fully incorporated. Stir in the chocolate chips with a spatula.

5.   Scoop the dough onto the prepared baking sheet.

6.   Place the baking sheet on the bake position.

7.   Select Bake, set temperature to 325°F (160°C), and set the time to 22 minutes.

8.	Bake until the cookies are golden brown.

9.	When cooking is complete, transfer the baking sheet onto a wire rack to cool completely before serving.

191..Fast Chocolate Cheesecake

Prep time: 5 minutes | Cook time: 18 minutes | Serves 6
Crust:
½ cup butter, melted
½ cup coconut flour
2 tablespoons stevia
Cooking spray
Topping:
4 ounces (113 g) unsweetened baker's chocolate
1 cup mascarpone cheese, at room temperature
1 teaspoon vanilla extract
2 drops peppermint extract

1.	Lightly coat a baking pan with cooking spray.

2.	In a mixing bowl, whisk together the flour, butter, and stevia until well combined. Transfer the mixture to the prepared baking pan.

3.	Place the pan on the bake position.

4.	Select Bake, set temperature to 350ºF (180ºC), and set time to 18 minutes.

5.	When done, a toothpick inserted in the center should come out clean.

6.	Remove the crust from the air fryer grill to a wire rack to cool.

7.	Once cooled completely, place it in the freezer for 20 minutes.

8.	When ready, combine all the ingredients for the topping in a small bowl and stir to incorporate.

9.	Spread this topping over the crust and let it sit for another 15 minutes in the freezer.

10.	Serve chilled.

192.Peach and Blueberry Tart

Prep time: 10 minutes | Cook time: 30 minutes | Serves 6 to 8
4 peaches, pitted and sliced
1 cup fresh blueberries
2 tablespoons cornstarch
3 tablespoons sugar
1 tablespoon freshly squeezed lemon juice
Cooking spray

1 sheet frozen puff pastry, thawed
1 tablespoon nonfat or low-fat milk
Confectioners' sugar, for dusting

1.	Add the blueberries, peaches, sugar, cornstarch, and lemon juice to a large bowl and toss to coat.

2.	Spritz a round baking pan with cooking spray.

3.	Unfold the pastry and put on the prepared baking pan.

4.	Lay the peach slices on the pan, slightly overlapping them. Scatter the blueberries over the peach.

5.	Drape the pastry over the outside of the fruit and press pleats firmly together. Brush the milk over the pastry.

6.	Place the pan on the bake position.

7.	Select Bake, set temperature to 400ºF (205ºC), and set time to 30 minutes.

8.	Bake until the crust is golden brown and the fruit is bubbling.

9.	When cooking is complete, remove the pan from the air fryer grill and allow to cool for 10 minutes.

10.	Serve the tart with the confectioners' sugar sprinkled on top.

Cinnamon Softened Apples

Prep time: 15 minutes | Cook time: 12 minutes | Serves 4
1 cup packed light brown sugar
2 teaspoons ground cinnamon
2 medium Granny Smith apples, peeled and diced

1.	Thoroughly combine the cinnamon and brown sugar in a medium bowl.

2.	Add the apples to the bowl and stir until well coated. Transfer the apples to a baking pan.

3.	Place the pan on the bake position.

4.	Select Bake, set temperature to 350ºF (180ºC), and set time to 12 minutes.

5.	After about 9 minutes, stir the apples and bake for an additional 3 minutes. When cooking is complete, the apples should be softened.

6.	Serve warm.

193.Berries with Nuts Streusel Topping

Prep time: 5 minutes | Cook time: 17 minutes | Serves 3

½ cup mixed berries
Cooking spray
Topping:
1 egg, beaten
3 tablespoons almonds, slivered
3 tablespoons chopped pecans
2 tablespoons chopped walnuts
3 tablespoons granulated Swerve
2 tablespoons cold salted butter, cut into pieces
½ teaspoon ground cinnamon

1. Lightly spray a baking dish with cooking spray.
2. Make the topping: In a medium bowl, stir together the beaten egg, nuts, butter, cinnamon, and Swerve until well blended.
3. Put the mixed berries in the bottom of the baking dish and spread the topping over the top.
4. Place the baking dish on the bake position.
5. Select Bake, set temperature to 340ºF (171ºC), and set time to 17 minutes.
6. When cooking is complete, the fruit should be bubbly and topping should be golden brown.
7. Allow to cool for 5 to 10 minutes before serving.

194.Golden Peach and Blueberry Galette

Prep time: 10 minutes | Cook time: 20 minutes | Serves 6

1 pint blueberries, rinsed and picked through (about 2 cups)
2 large peaches or nectarines, peeled and cut into ½-inch slices (about 2 cups)
$1/3$ cup plus 2 tablespoons granulated sugar, divided
2 tablespoons unbleached all-purpose flour
½ teaspoon grated lemon zest (optional)
¼ teaspoon ground allspice or cinnamon
Pinch kosher or fine salt
1 (9-inch) refrigerated piecrust (or use homemade)
2 teaspoons unsalted butter, cut into pea-size pieces
1 large egg, beaten

1. Mix together the peaches, blueberries, flour, $1/3$ cup of sugar, salt, allspice, and lemon zest (if desired) in a medium bowl.
2. Unroll the crust on the sheet pan, patching any tears if needed. Place the fruit in the center of the crust, leaving about 1½ inches of space around the edges. Scatter the butter pieces over the fruit. Fold the outside edge of the crust over the outer circle of the fruit, making pleats as needed.
3. Brush the egg over the crust. Sprinkle the crust and fruit with the remaining 2 tablespoons of sugar.
4. Place the pan on the bake position.
5. Select Bake, set temperature to 350ºF (180ºC), and set time to 20 minutes.
6. After about 15 minutes, check the galette, rotating the pan if the crust is not browning evenly. Continue cooking until the crust is deep golden brown and the fruit is bubbling.
7. When cooking is complete, remove the pan from the air fryer grill and allow to cool for 10 minutes before slicing and serving .

195..Coffee Cake

Prep time: 5 minutes | Cook time: 30 minutes | Serves 8
Dry Ingredients:
1½ cups almond flour
½ cup coconut meal
$2/3$ cup Swerve
1 teaspoon baking powder
¼ teaspoon salt
Wet Ingredients:
1 egg
1 stick butter, melted
½ cup hot strongly brewed coffee
Topping:
½ cup confectioner's Swerve
¼ cup coconut flour
3 tablespoons coconut oil
1 teaspoon ground cinnamon
½ teaspoon ground cardamom

1. In a medium bowl, combine the almond flour, salt, baking powder, coconut meal, and Swerve.
2. In a large bowl, whisk the melted butter, egg, and coffee until smooth.
3. Add the dry mixture to the wet and stir until well incorporated. Transfer the batter to a greased baking pan.
4. Stir together all the ingredients for the topping in a small bowl. Spread the topping over the batter and smooth the top with a spatula.
5. Place the pan on the bake position.

6. Select Bake, set temperature to 330ºF (166ºC), and set time to 30 minutes.
7. When cooking is complete, the cake should spring back when gently pressed with your fingers.
8. Rest for 10 minutes before serving.

196.Apple and Peach Crisp

Prep time: 10 minutes | Cook time: 10 to 12 minutes | Serves 4
2 peaches, peeled, pitted, and chopped
1 apple, peeled and chopped
2 tablespoons honey
3 tablespoons packed brown sugar
2 tablespoons unsalted butter, at room temperature
½ cup quick-cooking oatmeal
$^1/_3$ cup whole-wheat pastry flour
½ teaspoon ground cinnamon
1. Place the peaches, apple, and honey in a baking pan and toss until thoroughly combined.
2. Mix together the butter, pastry flour, brown sugar, oatmeal, and cinnamon in a medium bowl and stir until crumbly. Sprinkle this mixture generously on top of the peaches and apples.
3. Place the pan on the bake position.
4. Select Bake, set temperature to 380ºF (193ºC), and set the time to 10 minutes.
5. Bake until the fruit is bubbling and the topping is golden brown.
6. Once cooking is complete, remove the pan from the air fryer grill and allow to cool for 5 minutes before serving.

197.Cacio e Pepe Air-Fried Ravioli

Prep/Cook Time: 25 mins, Servings 10
Ingredients
- 1 (10-oz.) pkg. refrigerated cheese ravioli (such as Buitoni)
- 1 cup Italian-seasoned breadcrumbs
- 2 ounces Parmigiano-Reggiano cheese, grated (about 1/2 cup), divided
- 2 ounces pecorino Romano cheese, grated (about 1/2 cup), divided
- 1 ¼ teaspoons black pepper, divided
- 3 large eggs, lightly beaten
- 1 tablespoon chopped fresh flat-leaf parsley
- Warm marinara sauce, if desired
Instructions

- Cook ravioli in a pot of boiling water for 6 minutes. Drain and set aside on paper towels to dry.
- Stir together breadcrumbs, 1/3 cup of the Parmigiano Reggiano, 1/3 cup of the Pecorino, and 1 teaspoon of the black pepper in a shallow dish. Place eggs in a second shallow dish. Dip ravioli in egg, then dredge in bread crumb mixture, pressing to coat both sides.
- Working in batches, place ravioli in a single layer in basket of an air fryer lightly coated with cooking spray. Cook at 350°F for 7 minutes, turning once halfway through. Place air fried ravioli on a platter; sprinkle with parsley and remaining cheeses and pepper. Serve with marinara, if desired.

Nutrition Info : Calories 326 Calories from Fat 72, Protein 23g

198.Easy Chocolate and Coconut Cake

Prep time: 5 minutes | Cook time: 15 minutes | Serves 6
½ cup unsweetened chocolate, chopped
½ stick butter, at room temperature
1 tablespoon liquid stevia
1½ cups coconut flour
2 eggs, whisked
½ teaspoon vanilla extract
A pinch of fine sea salt
Cooking spray
1. Place the chocolate, stevia, and butter in a microwave-safe bowl. Microwave for about 30 seconds until melted.
2. Let the chocolate mixture cool for 5 to 10 minutes.
3. Add the remaining ingredients to the bowl of chocolate mixture and whisk to incorporate.
4. Lightly spray a baking pan with cooking spray.
5. Scrape the chocolate mixture into the prepared baking pan.
6. Place the pan on the bake position.
7. Select Bake, set temperature to 330ºF (166ºC), and set time to 15 minutes.
8. When cooking is complete, the top should spring back lightly when gently pressed with your fingers.
9. Let the cake cool for 5 minutes and serve.

199.Chocolate-Coconut Cake

Prep time: 5 minutes | Cook time: 15 minutes | Serves 10

1¼ cups unsweetened bakers' chocolate

1 stick butter

1 teaspoon liquid stevia

$^1/_3$ cup shredded coconut

2 tablespoons coconut milk

2 eggs, beaten

Cooking spray

1.   Lightly spritz a baking pan with cooking spray.

2.   Place the butter, chocolate, and stevia in a microwave-safe bowl. Microwave for about 30 seconds until melted. Let the chocolate mixture cool to room temperature.

3.   Add the remaining ingredients to the chocolate mixture and stir until well incorporated. Pour the batter into the prepared baking pan.

4.   Place the pan on the bake position.

5.   Select Bake, set temperature to 330ºF (166ºC), and set time to 15 minutes.

6.   When cooking is complete, a toothpick inserted in the center should come out clean.

7.   Remove from the air fryer grill and allow to cool for about 10 minutes before serving.

200.Classic Vanilla Pound Cake

Prep time: 5 minutes | Cook time: 30 minutes | Serves 8

1 stick butter, at room temperature

1 cup Swerve

4 eggs

1½ cups coconut flour

½ cup buttermilk

½ teaspoon baking soda

½ teaspoon baking powder

¼ teaspoon salt

1 teaspoon vanilla essence

A pinch of ground star anise

A pinch of freshly grated nutmeg

Cooking spray

1.   Spray a baking pan with cooking spray.

2.   With an electric mixer or hand mixer, beat the butter and Swerve until creamy. One at a time, mix in the eggs and whisk until fluffy. Add the remaining ingredients and stir to combine.

3.   Transfer the batter to the prepared baking pan.

4.   Place the pan on the bake position.

5.   Select Bake, set temperature to 320ºF (160ºC), and set time to 30 minutes. Rotate the pan halfway through the cooking time.

6.   When cooking is complete, the center of the cake should be springy.

7.   Allow the cake to cool in the pan for 10 minutes before removing and serving.

CHAPTER 10 CASSEROLES, FRITTATA, AND QUICHE

201.Cheesy Chicken Divan

Prep time: 5 minutes | Cook time: 24 minutes | Serves 4

4 chicken breasts
Salt and ground black pepper, to taste
1 head broccoli, cut into florets
½ cup cream of mushroom soup
1 cup shredded Cheddar cheese
½ cup croutons
Cooking spray

1. Spritz the air fry basket with cooking spray.
2. Put the chicken breasts in the air fry basket and sprinkle with salt and ground black pepper.
3. Place the basket on the air fry position.
4. Select Air Fry. Set temperature to 390ºF (199ºC) and set time to 14 minutes. Flip the breasts halfway through the cooking time.
5. When cooking is complete, the breasts should be well browned and tender.
6. Remove the breasts from the air fryer grill and allow to cool for a few minutes on a plate, then cut the breasts into bite-size pieces.
7. Combine the chicken, broccoli, mushroom soup, and Cheddar cheese in a large bowl. Stir to mix well.
8. Spritz a baking pan with cooking spray. Pour the chicken mixture into the pan. Spread the croutons over the mixture.
9. Place the pan on the bake position.
10. Select Bake. Set time to 10 minutes.
11. When cooking is complete, the croutons should be lightly browned and the mixture should be set.
12. Remove the baking pan from the air fryer grill and serve immediately.

202.Cheesy-Creamy Broccoli Casserole

Prep time: 5 minutes | Cook time: 30 minutes | Serves 6

4 cups broccoli florets
¼ cup heavy whipping cream
½ cup sharp Cheddar cheese, shredded
¼ cup ranch dressing
Kosher salt and ground black pepper, to taste

1. Combine all the ingredients in a large bowl. Toss to coat well broccoli well.
2. Pour the mixture into a baking pan.
3. Place the pan on the bake position.
4. Select Bake, set temperature to 375ºF (190ºC) and set time to 30 minutes.
5. When cooking is complete, the broccoli should be tender.
6. Remove the baking pan from the air fryer grill and serve immediately.

203.Cheesy Chorizo, Corn, and Potato Frittata

Prep time: 8 minutes | Cook time: 12 minutes | Serves 4

2 tablespoons olive oil
1 chorizo, sliced
4 eggs
½ cup corn
1 large potato, boiled and cubed
1 tablespoon chopped parsley
½ cup feta cheese, crumbled
Salt and ground black pepper, to taste

1. Heat the olive oil in a nonstick skillet over medium heat until shimmering.
2. Add the chorizo and cook for 4 minutes or until golden brown.
3. Whisk the eggs in a bowl, then sprinkle with salt and ground black pepper.
4. Mix the remaining ingredients in the egg mixture, then pour the chorizo and its fat into a baking pan. Pour in the egg mixture.
5. Place the pan on the bake position.
6. Select Bake, set temperature to 330ºF (166ºC) and set time to 8 minutes. Stir the mixture halfway through.
7. When cooking is complete, the eggs should be set.
8. Serve immediately.

204.Taco Beef and Green Chile Casserole

Prep time: 10 minutes | Cook time: 15 minutes | Serves 4

1 pound (454 g) 85% lean ground beef
1 tablespoon taco seasoning

1 (7-ounce / 198-g) can diced mild green chiles
½ cup milk
2 large eggs
1 cup shredded Mexican cheese blend
2 tablespoons all-purpose flour
½ teaspoon kosher salt
Cooking spray

1.   Spritz a baking pan with cooking spray.
2.   Toss the ground beef with taco seasoning in a large bowl to mix well. Pour the seasoned ground beef in the prepared baking pan.
3.   Combing the remaining ingredients in a medium bowl. Whisk to mix well, then pour the mixture over the ground beef.
4.   Place the pan on the bake position.
5.   Select Bake, set temperature to 350ºF (180ºC) and set time to 15 minutes.
6.   When cooking is complete, a toothpick inserted in the center should come out clean.
7.   Remove the casserole from the air fryer grill and allow to cool for 5 minutes, then slice to serve.

205..Golden Asparagus Frittata

Prep time: 5 minutes | Cook time: 25 minutes | Serves 2 to 4

1 cup asparagus spears, cut into 1-inch pieces
1 teaspoon vegetable oil
1 tablespoon milk
6 eggs, beaten
2 ounces (57 g) goat cheese, crumbled
1 tablespoon minced chives, optional
Kosher salt and pepper, to taste

1.   Add the asparagus spears to a small bowl and drizzle with the vegetable oil. Toss until well coated and transfer to the air fry basket.
2.   Place the basket on the air fry position.
3.   Select Air Fry. Set temperature to 400ºF (205ºC) and set time to 5 minutes. Flip the asparagus halfway through.
4.   When cooking is complete, the asparagus should be tender and slightly wilted.
5.   Remove the asparagus from the air fryer grill to a baking pan.
6.   Stir together the milk and eggs in a medium bowl. Pour the mixture over the asparagus in the pan.

Sprinkle with the goat cheese and the chives (if using) over the eggs. Season with salt and pepper.
7.   Place the pan on the bake position.
8.   Select Bake, set temperature to 320ºF (160ºC) and set time to 20 minutes.
9.   When cooking is complete, the top should be golden and the eggs should be set.
10.   Transfer to a serving dish. Slice and serve.

206..Corn and Bell Pepper Casserole

Prep time: 10 minutes | Cook time: 20 minutes | Serves 4

1 cup corn kernels
¼ cup bell pepper, finely chopped
½ cup low-fat milk
1 large egg, beaten
½ cup yellow cornmeal
½ cup all-purpose flour
½ teaspoon baking powder
2 tablespoons melted unsalted butter
1 tablespoon granulated sugar
Pinch of cayenne pepper
¼ teaspoon kosher salt
Cooking spray

1.   Spritz a baking pan with cooking spray.
2.   Combine all the ingredients in a large bowl. Stir to mix well. Pour the mixture into the baking pan.
3.   Place the pan on the bake position.
4.   Select Bake, set temperature to 330ºF (166ºC) and set time to 20 minutes.
5.   When cooking is complete, the casserole should be lightly browned and set.
6.   Remove the baking pan from the air fryer grill and serve immediately.

207..Creamy-Mustard Pork Gratin

Prep time: 15 minutes | Cook time: 21 minutes | Serves 4

2 tablespoons olive oil
2 pounds (907 g) pork tenderloin, cut into serving-size pieces
1 teaspoon dried marjoram
¼ teaspoon chili powder
1 teaspoon coarse sea salt
½ teaspoon freshly ground black pepper
1 cup Ricotta cheese
1½ cups chicken broth

76

1 tablespoon mustard
Cooking spray

1. Spritz a baking pan with cooking spray.
2. Heat the olive oil in a nonstick skillet over medium-high heat until shimmering.
3. Add the pork and sauté for 6 minutes or until lightly browned.
4. Transfer the pork to the prepared baking pan and sprinkle with marjoram, salt, chili powder, and ground black pepper.
5. Combine the remaining ingredients in a large bowl. Stir to mix well. Pour the mixture over the pork in the pan.
6. Place the pan on the bake position.
7. Select Bake, set temperature to 350ºF (180ºC) and set time to 15 minutes. Stir the mixture halfway through.
8. When cooking is complete, the mixture should be frothy and the cheese should be melted.
9. Serve immediately.

208..Broccoli, Carrot, and Tomato Quiche

Prep time: 6 minutes | Cook time: 14 minutes | Serves 4

4 eggs
1 teaspoon dried thyme
1 cup whole milk
1 steamed carrots, diced
2 cups steamed broccoli florets
2 medium tomatoes, diced
¼ cup crumbled feta cheese
1 cup grated Cheddar cheese
1 teaspoon chopped parsley
Salt and ground black pepper, to taste
Cooking spray

1. Spritz a baking pan with cooking spray.
2. Whisk together the eggs, salt, thyme, and ground black pepper in a bowl and fold in the milk while mixing.
3. Put the broccoli, carrots, and tomatoes in the prepared baking pan, then spread with ½ cup Cheddar cheese and feta cheese. Pour the egg mixture over, then scatter with remaining Cheddar on top.
4. Place the pan on the bake position.
5. Select Bake, set temperature to 350ºF (180ºC) and set time to 14 minutes.

6. When cooking is complete, the egg should be set and the quiche should be puffed.
7. Remove the quiche from the air fryer grill and top with chopped parsley, then slice to serve.

209.Herbed Cheddar Cheese Frittata

Prep time: 10 minutes | Cook time: 20 minutes | Serves 4

½ cup shredded Cheddar cheese
½ cup half-and-half
4 large eggs
2 tablespoons chopped scallion greens
2 tablespoons chopped fresh parsley
½ teaspoon kosher salt
½ teaspoon ground black pepper
Cooking spray

1. Spritz a baking pan with cooking spray.
2. Whisk together all the ingredients in a large bowl, then pour the mixture into the prepared baking pan.
3. Place the pan on the bake position.
4. Select Bake, set temperature to 300ºF (150ºC) and set time to 20 minutes. Stir the mixture halfway through.
5. When cooking is complete, the eggs should be set.
6. Serve immediately.

210.Cauliflower, Okra, and Pepper Casserole

Prep time: 8 minutes | Cook time: 12 minutes | Serves 4

1 head cauliflower, cut into florets
1 cup okra, chopped
1 yellow bell pepper, chopped
2 eggs, beaten
½ cup chopped onion
1 tablespoon soy sauce
2 tablespoons olive oil
Salt and ground black pepper, to taste

1. Spritz a baking pan with cooking spray.
2. Put the cauliflower in a food processor and pulse to rice the cauliflower.
3. Pour the cauliflower rice in the baking pan and add the remaining ingredients. Stir to mix well.
4. Place the pan on the bake position.

5.   Select Bake, set temperature to 380ºF (193ºC) and set time to 12 minutes.

6.   When cooking is complete, the eggs should be set.

7.   Remove the baking pan from the air fryer grill and serve immediately.

211. Sumptuous Chicken and Vegetable Casserole

Prep time: 15 minutes | Cook time: 15 minutes | Serves 4

4 boneless and skinless chicken breasts, cut into cubes
2 carrots, sliced
1 yellow bell pepper, cut into strips
1 red bell pepper, cut into strips
15 ounces (425 g) broccoli florets
1 cup snow peas
1 scallion, sliced
Cooking spray
Sauce:
1 teaspoon Sriracha
3 tablespoons soy sauce
2 tablespoons oyster sauce
1 tablespoon rice wine vinegar
1 teaspoon cornstarch
1 tablespoon grated ginger
2 garlic cloves, minced
1 teaspoon sesame oil
1 tablespoon brown sugar

1.   Spritz a baking pan with cooking spray.

2.   Combine the chicken, bell peppers, and carrot in a large bowl. Stir to mix well.

3.   Combine the ingredients for the sauce in a separate bowl. Stir to mix well.

4.   Pour the chicken mixture into the baking pan, then pour the sauce over. Stir to coat well.

5.   Place the pan on the bake position.

6.   Select Bake, set temperature to 370ºF (188ºC) and set time to 13 minutes. Add the broccoli and snow peas to the pan halfway through.

7.   When cooking is complete, the vegetables should be tender.

8.   Remove the pan from the air fryer grill and sprinkle with sliced scallion before serving.

212. Easy Chickpea and Spinach Casserole

Prep time: 10 minutes | Cook time: 21 to 22 minutes | Serves 4

2 tablespoons olive oil
2 garlic cloves, minced
1 tablespoon ginger, minced
1 onion, chopped
1 chili pepper, minced
Salt and ground black pepper, to taste
1 pound (454 g) spinach
1 can coconut milk
½ cup dried tomatoes, chopped
1 (14-ounce / 397-g) can chickpeas, drained

1.   Heat the olive oil in a saucepan over medium heat. Sauté the ginger and garlic in the olive oil for 1 minute, or until fragrant.

2.   Add the chili pepper, onion, salt and pepper to the saucepan. Sauté for 3 minutes.

3.   Mix in the spinach and sauté for 3 to 4 minutes or until the vegetables become soft. Remove from heat.

4.   Pour the vegetable mixture into a baking pan. Stir in chickpeas, dried tomatoes and coconut milk until well blended.

5.   Place the pan on the bake position.

6.   Select Bake, set temperature to 370ºF (188ºC) and set time to 15 minutes.

7.   When cooking is complete, transfer the casserole to a serving dish. Let cool for 5 minutes before serving.

213. Classic Mediterranean Quiche

Prep time: 10 minutes | Cook time: 30 minutes | Serves 4

4 eggs
¼ cup chopped Kalamata olives
½ cup chopped tomatoes
¼ cup chopped onion
½ cup milk
1 cup crumbled feta cheese
½ tablespoon chopped oregano
½ tablespoon chopped basil
Salt and ground black pepper, to taste
Cooking spray

1.   Spritz a baking pan with cooking spray.

2.   Whisk the eggs with remaining ingredients in a large bowl. Stir to mix well.

3. Pour the mixture into the prepared baking pan.

4. Place the pan on the bake position.

5. Select Bake, set temperature to 340ºF (171ºC) and set time to 30 minutes.

6. When cooking is complete, the eggs should be set and a toothpick inserted in the center should come out clean.

7. Serve immediately.

214.Cheesy Mushrooms and Spinach Frittata

Prep time: 7 minutes | Cook time: 8 minutes | Serves 2

1 cup chopped mushrooms
2 cups spinach, chopped
4 eggs, lightly beaten
3 ounces (85 g) feta cheese, crumbled
2 tablespoons heavy cream
A handful of fresh parsley, chopped
Salt and ground black pepper, to taste
Cooking spray

1. Spritz a baking pan with cooking spray.

2. Whisk together all the ingredients in a large bowl. Stir to mix well.

3. Pour the mixture in the prepared baking pan.

4. Place the pan on the bake position.

5. Select Bake, set temperature to 350ºF (180ºC) and set time to 8 minutes. Stir the mixture halfway through.

6. When cooking is complete, the eggs should be set.

7. Serve immediately.

215..Cheesy Asparagus and Grits Casserole

Prep time: 5 minutes | Cook time: 30 minutes | Serves 4

10 fresh asparagus spears, cut into 1-inch pieces
2 cups cooked grits, cooled to room temperature
2 teaspoons Worcestershire sauce
1 egg, beaten
½ teaspoon garlic powder
¼ teaspoon salt
2 slices provolone cheese, crushed
Cooking spray

1. Spritz a baking pan with cooking spray.

2. Set the asparagus in the air fry basket. Spritz the asparagus with cooking spray.

3. Place the basket on the air fry position.

4. Select Air Fry. Set temperature to 390ºF (199ºC) and set time to 5 minutes. Flip the asparagus halfway through.

5. When cooking is complete, the asparagus should be lightly browned and crispy.

6. Meanwhile, combine the grits, egg, salt, garlic powder, and Worcestershire sauce in a bowl. Stir to mix well.

7. Pour half of the grits mixture in the prepared baking pan, then spread with fried asparagus.

8. Spread the cheese over the asparagus and pour the remaining grits over.

9. Place the pan on the bake position.

10. Select Bake. Set time to 25 minutes.

11. When cooking is complete, the egg should be set.

12. Serve immediately.

216.Cauliflower Florets and Pumpkin Casserole

Prep time: 15 minutes | Cook time: 50 minutes | Serves 6

1 cup chicken broth
2 cups cauliflower florets
1 cup canned pumpkin purée
¼ cup heavy cream
1 teaspoon vanilla extract
2 large eggs, beaten
$^1/_3$ cup unsalted butter, melted, plus more for greasing the pan
¼ cup sugar
1 teaspoon fine sea salt
Chopped fresh parsley leaves, for garnish
TOPPING:
½ cup blanched almond flour
1 cup chopped pecans
$^1/_3$ cup unsalted butter, melted
½ cup sugar

1. Pour the chicken broth in a baking pan, then add the cauliflower.

2. Place the pan on the bake position.

3.   Select Bake, set temperature to 350ºF (180ºC) and set time to 20 minutes.

4.   When cooking is complete, the cauliflower should be soft.

5.   Meanwhile, combine the ingredients for the topping in a large bowl. Stir to mix well.

6.   Pat the cauliflower dry with paper towels, then place in a food processor and pulse with heavy cream, pumpkin purée, eggs, butter, sugar, vanilla extract, and salt until smooth.

7.   Clean the baking pan and grease with more butter, then pour the purée mixture in the pan. Spread the topping over the mixture.

8.   Place the baking pan back to the air fryer grill. Select Bake and set time to 30 minutes.

9.   When baking is complete, the topping of the casserole should be lightly browned.

10.   Remove the casserole from the air fryer grill and serve with fresh parsley on top.

217..Cheesy-Creamy Green Bean Casserole

Prep time: 4 minutes | Cook time: 6 minutes | Serves 4

1 tablespoon melted butter
1 cup green beans
6 ounces (170 g) Cheddar cheese, shredded
7 ounces (198 g) Parmesan cheese, shredded
¼ cup heavy cream
Sea salt, to taste

1.   Grease a baking pan with the melted butter.

2.   Add the green beans, black pepper, salt, and Cheddar to the prepared baking pan. Stir to mix well, then spread the Parmesan and cream on top.

3.   Place the pan on the bake position.

4.   Select Bake, set temperature to 400ºF (205ºC) and set time to 6 minutes.

5.   When cooking is complete, the beans should be tender and the cheese should be melted.

6.   Serve immediately.

CHAPTER 11 WRAPS AND SANDWICHES

218..Crunchy Chicken Egg Rolls

Prep time: 10 minutes | Cook time: 23 to 24 minutes | Serves 4

1 pound (454 g) ground chicken
2 teaspoons olive oil
2 garlic cloves, minced
1 teaspoon grated fresh ginger
2 cups white cabbage, shredded
1 onion, chopped
¼ cup soy sauce
8 egg roll wrappers
1 egg, beaten
Cooking spray

1.   Spritz the air fry basket with cooking spray.
2.   Heat olive oil in a saucepan over medium heat. Sauté the garlic and ginger in the olive oil for 1 minute, or until fragrant. Add the ground chicken to the saucepan. Sauté for 5 minutes, or until the chicken is cooked through. Add the cabbage, onion and soy sauce and sauté for 5 to 6 minutes, or until the vegetables become soft. Remove the saucepan from the heat.
3.   Unfold the egg roll wrappers on a clean work surface. Divide the chicken mixture among the wrappers and brush the edges of the wrappers with the beaten egg. Tightly roll up the egg rolls, enclosing the filling. Arrange the rolls in the basket.
4.   Place the basket on the air fry position.
5.   Select Air Fry, set temperature to 370ºF (188ºC) and set time to 12 minutes. Flip the rolls halfway through the cooking time.
6.   When cooked, the rolls will be crispy and golden brown.
7.   Transfer to a platter and let cool for 5 minutes before serving.

219..Panko-Crusted Avocado and Slaw Tacos

Prep time: 15 minutes | Cook time: 6 minutes | Serves 4

¼ cup all-purpose flour
¼ teaspoon salt, plus more as needed
¼ teaspoon ground black pepper
2 large egg whites
1¼ cups panko bread crumbs
2 tablespoons olive oil
2 avocados, peeled and halved, cut into ½-inch-thick slices
½ small red cabbage, thinly sliced
1 deseeded jalapeño, thinly sliced
2 green onions, thinly sliced
½ cup cilantro leaves
¼ cup mayonnaise
Juice and zest of 1 lime
4 corn tortillas, warmed
½ cup sour cream
Cooking spray

1.   Spritz the air fry basket with cooking spray.
2.   Pour the flour in a large bowl and sprinkle with salt and black pepper, then stir to mix well.
3.   Whisk the egg whites in a separate bowl. Combine the panko with olive oil on a shallow dish.
4.   Dredge the avocado slices in the bowl of flour, then into the egg to coat. Shake the excess off, then roll the slices over the panko.
5.   Arrange the avocado slices in a single layer in the basket and spritz the cooking spray.
6.   Place the basket on the air fry position.
7.   Select Air Fry, set temperature to 400ºF (205ºC) and set time to 6 minutes. Flip the slices halfway through with tongs.
8.   When cooking is complete, the avocado slices should be tender and lightly browned.
9.   Combine the cabbage, onions, jalapeño, cilantro leaves, lime juice, mayo, and zest, and a touch of salt in a separate large bowl. Toss to mix well.
10.   Unfold the tortillas on a clean work surface, then spread with cabbage slaw and air fried avocados. Top with sour cream and serve.

220.Golden Baja Fish Tacos

Prep time: 15 minutes | Cook time: 17 minutes | Makes 6 tacos

1 egg
5 ounces (142 g) Mexican beer
¾ cup all-purpose flour
¾ cup cornstarch

¼ teaspoon chili powder

½ teaspoon ground cumin

½ pound (227 g) cod, cut into large pieces

6 corn tortillas

Cooking spray

Salsa:

1 mango, peeled and diced

¼ red bell pepper, diced

½ small jalapeño, diced

¼ red onion, minced

Juice of half a lime

Pinch chopped fresh cilantro

¼ teaspoon salt

¼ teaspoon ground black pepper

1. Spritz the air fry basket with cooking spray.

2. Whisk the egg with beer in a bowl. Combine the flour, chili powder, cumin, and cornstarch in a separate bowl.

3. Dredge the cod in the egg mixture first, then in the flour mixture to coat well. Shake the excess off.

4. Arrange the cod in the air fry basket and spritz with cooking spray.

5. Place the basket on the air fry position.

6. Select Air Fry, set temperature to 380ºF (193ºC) and set time to 17 minutes. Flip the cod halfway through the cooking time.

7. When cooked, the cod should be golden brown and crunchy.

8. Meanwhile, combine the ingredients for the salsa in a small bowl. Stir to mix well.

9. Unfold the tortillas on a clean work surface, then divide the fish on the tortillas and spread the salsa on top. Fold to serve.

221.Golden Cabbage and Mushroom Spring Rolls

Prep time: 20 minutes | Cook time: 14 minutes | Makes 14 spring rolls

2 tablespoons vegetable oil

4 cups sliced Napa cabbage

5 ounces (142 g) shiitake mushrooms, diced

3 carrots, cut into thin matchsticks

1 tablespoon minced fresh ginger

1 tablespoon minced garlic

1 bunch scallions, white and light green parts only, sliced

2 tablespoons soy sauce

1 (4-ounce / 113-g) package cellophane noodles

¼ teaspoon cornstarch

1 (12-ounce / 340-g) package frozen spring roll wrappers, thawed

Cooking spray

1. Heat the olive oil in a nonstick skillet over medium-high heat until shimmering.

2. Add the cabbage, carrots, and mushrooms and sauté for 3 minutes or until tender.

3. Add the garlic, scallions, and ginger and sauté for 1 minutes or until fragrant.

4. Mix in the soy sauce and turn off the heat. Discard any liquid remains in the skillet and allow to cool for a few minutes.

5. Bring a pot of water to a boil, then turn off the heat and pour in the noodles. Let sit for 10 minutes or until the noodles are al dente. Transfer 1 cup of the noodles in the skillet and toss with the cooked vegetables. Reserve the remaining noodles for other use.

6. Dissolve the cornstarch in a small dish of water, then place the wrappers on a clean work surface. Dab the edges of the wrappers with cornstarch.

7. Scoop up 3 tablespoons of filling in the center of each wrapper, then fold the corner in front of you over the filling. Tuck the wrapper under the filling, then fold the corners on both sides into the center. Keep rolling to seal the wrapper. Repeat with remaining wrappers.

8. Spritz the air fry basket with cooking spray. Arrange the wrappers in the basket and spritz with cooking spray.

9. Place the basket on the air fry position.

10. Select Air Fry, set temperature to 400ºF (205ºC) and set time to 10 minutes. Flip the wrappers halfway through the cooking time.

11. When cooking is complete, the wrappers will be golden brown.

12. Serve immediately.

222.Cheesy Philly Steaks

Prep time: 20 minutes | Cook time: 20 minutes | Serves 2

12 ounces (340 g) boneless rib-eye steak, sliced thinly

½ teaspoon Worcestershire sauce

½ teaspoon soy sauce

Kosher salt and ground black pepper, to taste

½ green bell pepper, stemmed, deseeded, and thinly sliced

½ small onion, halved and thinly sliced

1 tablespoon vegetable oil

2 soft hoagie rolls, split three-fourths of the way through

1 tablespoon butter, softened

2 slices provolone cheese, halved

1. Combine the steak, soy sauce, salt, ground black pepper, and Worcestershire sauce in a large bowl. Toss to coat well. Set aside.

2. Combine the bell pepper, onion, vegetable oil, salt, and ground black pepper in a separate bowl. Toss to coat the vegetables well.

3. Pour the steak and vegetables in the air fry basket.

4. Place the basket on the air fry position.

5. Select Air Fry, set temperature to 400°F (205°C) and set time to 15 minutes.

6. When cooked, the steak will be browned and vegetables will be tender. Transfer them on a plate. Set aside.

7. Brush the hoagie rolls with butter and place in the basket.

8. Select Toast and set time to 3 minutes. Place the basket on the toast position. When done, the rolls should be lightly browned.

9. Transfer the rolls to a clean work surface and divide the steak and vegetable mix in between the rolls. Spread with cheese. Place the stuffed rolls back in the basket.

10. Place the basket on the air fry position.

11. Select Air Fry and set time to 2 minutes. When done, the cheese should be melted.

12. Serve immediately.

223.Cheesy Chicken Wraps

Prep time: 30 minutes | Cook time: 5 minutes | Serves 12

2 large-sized chicken breasts, cooked and shredded

2 spring onions, chopped

10 ounces (284 g) Ricotta cheese

1 tablespoon rice vinegar

1 tablespoon molasses

1 teaspoon grated fresh ginger

¼ cup soy sauce

$1/3$ teaspoon sea salt

¼ teaspoon ground black pepper, or more to taste

48 wonton wrappers

Cooking spray

1. Spritz the air fry basket with cooking spray.

2. Combine all the ingredients, except for the wrappers in a large bowl. Toss to mix well.

3. Unfold the wrappers on a clean work surface, then divide and spoon the mixture in the middle of the wrappers.

4. Dab a little water on the edges of the wrappers, then fold the edge close to you over the filling. Tuck the edge under the filling and roll up to seal.

5. Arrange the wraps in the basket.

6. Place the basket on the air fry position.

7. Select Air Fry, set temperature to 375°F (190°C) and set time to 5 minutes. Flip the wraps halfway through the cooking time.

8. When cooking is complete, the wraps should be lightly browned.

9. Serve immediately.

224.Golden Avocado and Tomato Egg Rolls

Prep time: 10 minutes | Cook time: 5 minutes | Serves 5

10 egg roll wrappers

3 avocados, peeled and pitted

1 tomato, diced

Salt and ground black pepper, to taste

Cooking spray

1. Spritz the air fry basket with cooking spray.

2. Put the avocados and tomato in a food processor. Sprinkle with salt and ground black pepper. Pulse to mix and coarsely mash until smooth.

3. Unfold the wrappers on a clean work surface, then divide the mixture in the center of each wrapper. Roll the wrapper up and press to seal.

4. Transfer the rolls to the basket and spritz with cooking spray.

5. Place the basket on the air fry position.

6. Select Air Fry, set temperature to 350°F (180°C) and set time to 5 minutes. Flip the rolls halfway through the cooking time.

7. When cooked, the rolls should be golden brown.

8.   Serve immediately.

225.Korean Beef and Onion Tacos

Prep time: 1 hour 15 minutes | Cook time: 12 minutes | Serves 6

2 tablespoons gochujang
1 tablespoon soy sauce
2 tablespoons sesame seeds
2 teaspoons minced fresh ginger
2 cloves garlic, minced
2 tablespoons toasted sesame oil
2 teaspoons sugar
½ teaspoon kosher salt
1½ pounds (680 g) thinly sliced beef chuck
1 medium red onion, sliced
6 corn tortillas, warmed
¼ cup chopped fresh cilantro
½ cup kimchi
½ cup chopped green onions

1.   Combine the ginger, garlic, gochujang, sesame seeds, soy sauce, sesame oil, salt, and sugar in a large bowl. Stir to mix well.
2.   Dunk the beef chunk in the large bowl. Press to submerge, then wrap the bowl in plastic and refrigerate to marinate for at least 1 hour.
3.   Remove the beef chunk from the marinade and transfer to the air fry basket. Add the onion to the basket.
4.   Place the basket on the air fry position.
5.   Select Air Fry, set temperature to 400ºF (205ºC) and set time to 12 minutes. Stir the mixture halfway through the cooking time.
6.   When cooked, the beef will be well browned.
7.   Unfold the tortillas on a clean work surface, then divide the fried beef and onion on the tortillas. Spread the green onions, kimchi, and cilantro on top.
8.   Serve immediately.

226..Crispy Pea and Potato Samosas

Prep time: 30 minutes | Cook time: 22 minutes | Makes 16 samosas
Dough:
4 cups all-purpose flour, plus more for flouring the work surface
¼ cup plain yogurt
½ cup cold unsalted butter, cut into cubes
2 teaspoons kosher salt
1 cup ice water
Filling:
2 tablespoons vegetable oil
1 onion, diced
1½ teaspoons coriander
1½ teaspoons cumin
1 clove garlic, minced
1 teaspoon turmeric
1 teaspoon kosher salt
½ cup peas, thawed if frozen
2 cups mashed potatoes
2 tablespoons yogurt
Cooking spray
Chutney:
1 cup mint leaves, lightly packed
2 cups cilantro leaves, lightly packed
1 green chile pepper, deseeded and minced
½ cup minced onion
Juice of 1 lime
1 teaspoon granulated sugar
1 teaspoon kosher salt
2 tablespoons vegetable oil

1.   Put the flour, butter, salt, and yogurt in a food processor. Pulse to combine until grainy. Pour in the water and pulse until a smooth and firm dough forms.
2.   Transfer the dough on a clean and lightly floured working surface. Knead the dough and shape it into a ball. Cut in half and flatten the halves into 2 discs. Wrap them in plastic and let sit in refrigerator until ready to use.
3.   Meanwhile, make the filling: Heat the vegetable oil in a saucepan over medium heat.
4.   Add the onion and sauté for 5 minutes or until lightly browned.
5.   Add the coriander, garlic, cumin, salt, and turmeric and sauté for 2 minutes or until fragrant.
6.   Add the potatoes, peas, and yogurt and stir to combine well. Turn off the heat and allow to cool.
7.   Meanwhile, combine the ingredients for the chutney in a food processor. Pulse to mix well until glossy. Pour the chutney in a bowl and refrigerate until ready to use.
8.   Make the samosas: Remove the dough discs from the refrigerator and cut each disc into 8 parts. Shape each part into a ball, then roll the ball into a 6-

inch circle. Cut the circle in half and roll each half into a cone.

9. Scoop up 2 tablespoons of the filling into the cone, press the edges of the cone to seal and form into a triangle. Repeat with remaining dough and filling.

10. Spritz the air fry basket with cooking spray. Arrange the samosas in the basket and spritz with cooking spray.

11. Place the basket on the air fry position.

12. Select Air Fry, set temperature to 360ºF (182ºC) and set time to 15 minutes. Flip the samosas halfway through the cooking time.

13. When cooked, the samosas will be golden brown and crispy.

14. Serve the samosas with the chutney.

227..Cheesy Sweet Potato and Bean Burritos

Prep time: 15 minutes | Cook time: 30 minutes | Makes 6 burritos

2 sweet potatoes, peeled and cut into a small dice
1 tablespoon vegetable oil
Kosher salt and ground black pepper, to taste
6 large flour tortillas
1 (16-ounce / 454-g) can refried black beans, divided
1½ cups baby spinach, divided
6 eggs, scrambled
¾ cup grated Cheddar cheese, divided
¼ cup salsa
¼ cup sour cream
Cooking spray

1. Put the sweet potatoes in a large bowl, then drizzle with vegetable oil and sprinkle with salt and black pepper. Toss to coat well.

2. Place the potatoes in the air fry basket.

3. Place the basket on the air fry position.

4. Select Air Fry, set temperature to 400ºF (205ºC) and set time to 10 minutes. Flip the potatoes halfway through the cooking time.

5. When done, the potatoes should be lightly browned. Remove the potatoes from the air fryer grill.

6. Unfold the tortillas on a clean work surface. Divide the air fried sweet potatoes, black beans,

spinach, scrambled eggs, and cheese on top of the tortillas.

7. Fold the long side of the tortillas over the filling, then fold in the shorter side to wrap the filling to make the burritos.

8. Wrap the burritos in the aluminum foil and put in the basket.

9. Place the basket on the air fry position.

10. Select Air Fry, set temperature to 350ºF (180ºC) and set time to 20 minutes. Flip the burritos halfway through the cooking time.

11. Remove the burritos from the air fryer grill and spread with sour cream and salsa. Serve immediately.

228.Golden Chicken and Yogurt Taquitos

Prep time: 15 minutes | Cook time: 12 minutes | Serves 4

1 cup cooked chicken, shredded
¼ cup Greek yogurt
¼ cup salsa
1 cup shredded Mozzarella cheese
Salt and ground black pepper, to taste
4 flour tortillas
Cooking spray

1. Spritz the air fry basket with cooking spray.

2. Combine all the ingredients, except for the tortillas, in a large bowl. Stir to mix well.

3. Make the taquitos: Unfold the tortillas on a clean work surface, then scoop up 2 tablespoons of the chicken mixture in the middle of each tortilla. Roll the tortillas up to wrap the filling.

4. Arrange the taquitos in the basket and spritz with cooking spray.

5. Place the basket on the air fry position.

6. Select Air Fry, set temperature to 380ºF (193ºC) and set time to 12 minutes. Flip the taquitos halfway through the cooking time.

7. When cooked, the taquitos should be golden brown and the cheese should be melted.

8. Serve immediately.

229.Turkey Patties with Chive Mayo

Prep time: 10 minutes | Cook time: 15 minutes | Serves 6

12 burger buns

Cooking spray

Turkey Sliders:

¾ pound (340 g) turkey, minced

1 tablespoon oyster sauce

¼ cup pickled jalapeno, chopped

2 tablespoons chopped scallions

1 tablespoon chopped fresh cilantro

1 to 2 cloves garlic, minced

Sea salt and ground black pepper, to taste

Chive Mayo:

1 tablespoon chives

1 cup mayonnaise

Zest of 1 lime

1 teaspoon salt

1.   Spritz the air fry basket with cooking spray.

2.   Combine the ingredients for the turkey sliders in a large bowl. Stir to mix well. Shape the mixture into 6 balls, then bash the balls into patties.

3.   Arrange the patties in the basket and spritz with cooking spray.

4.   Place the basket on the air fry position.

5.   Select Air Fry, set temperature to 365ºF (185ºC) and set time to 15 minutes. Flip the patties halfway through the cooking time.

6.   Meanwhile, combine the ingredients for the chive mayo in a small bowl. Stir to mix well.

7.   When cooked, the patties will be well browned.

8.   Smear the patties with chive mayo, then assemble the patties between two buns to make the sliders. Serve immediately.

230.Crunchy Shrimp and Zucchini Potstickers

Prep time: 35 minutes | Cook time: 5 minutes | Serves 10

½ pound (227 g) peeled and deveined shrimp, finely chopped

1 medium zucchini, coarsely grated

1 tablespoon fish sauce

1 tablespoon green curry paste

2 scallions, thinly sliced

¼ cup basil, chopped

30 round dumpling wrappers

Cooking spray

1.   Combine the zucchini, chopped shrimp, curry paste, fish sauce, basil, and scallions in a large bowl. Stir to mix well.

2.   Unfold the dumpling wrappers on a clean work surface, dab a little water around the edges of each wrapper, then scoop up 1 teaspoon of filling in the middle of each wrapper.

3.   Make the potstickers: Fold the wrappers in half and press the edges to seal.

4.   Spritz the air fry basket with cooking spray.

5.   Transfer the potstickers to the basket and spritz with cooking spray.

6.   Place the basket on the air fry position.

7.   Select Air Fry, set temperature to 350ºF (180ºC) and set time to 5 minutes. Flip the potstickers halfway through the cooking time.

8.   When cooking is complete, the potstickers should be crunchy and lightly browned.

9.   Serve immediately.

231.Cod Tacos with Salsa

Prep time: 5 minutes | Cook time: 15 minutes | Serves 4

2 eggs

1¼ cups Mexican beer

1½ cups coconut flour

1½ cups almond flour

½ tablespoon chili powder

1 tablespoon cumin

Salt, to taste

1 pound (454 g) cod fillet, slice into large pieces

4 toasted corn tortillas

4 large lettuce leaves, chopped

¼ cup salsa

Cooking spray

1.   Spritz the air fry basket with cooking spray.

2.   Break the eggs in a bowl, then pour in the beer. Whisk to combine well.

3.   Combine the almond flour, coconut flour, cumin, chili powder, and salt in a separate bowl. Stir to mix well.

4.   Dunk the cod pieces in the egg mixture, then shake the excess off and dredge into the flour mixture to coat well. Arrange the cod in the basket.

5. Place the basket on the air fry position.

6. Select Air Fry, set temperature to 375ºF (190ºC) and set time to 15 minutes. Flip the cod halfway through the cooking time.

7. When cooking is complete, the cod should be golden brown.

8. Unwrap the toasted tortillas on a large plate, then divide the cod and lettuce leaves on top. Baste with salsa and wrap to serve.

232.Golden Spring Rolls

Prep time: 10 minutes | Cook time: 18 minutes | Serves 4

4 spring roll wrappers
½ cup cooked vermicelli noodles
1 teaspoon sesame oil
1 tablespoon freshly minced ginger
1 tablespoon soy sauce
1 clove garlic, minced
½ red bell pepper, deseeded and chopped
½ cup chopped carrot
½ cup chopped mushrooms
¼ cup chopped scallions
Cooking spray

1. Spritz the air fry basket with cooking spray and set aside.

2. Heat the sesame oil in a saucepan on medium heat. Sauté the garlic and ginger in the sesame oil for 1 minute, or until fragrant. Add soy sauce, carrot, red bell pepper, mushrooms and scallions. Sauté for 5 minutes or until the vegetables become tender. Mix in vermicelli noodles. Turn off the heat and remove them from the saucepan. Allow to cool for 10 minutes.

3. Lay out one spring roll wrapper with a corner pointed toward you. Scoop the noodle mixture on spring roll wrapper and fold corner up over the mixture. Fold left and right corners toward the center and continue to roll to make firmly sealed rolls.

4. Arrange the spring rolls in the basket and spritz with cooking spray.

5. Place the basket on the air fry position.

6. Select Air Fry, set temperature to 340ºF (171ºC) and set time to 12 minutes. Flip the spring rolls halfway through the cooking time.

7. When done, the spring rolls will be golden brown and crispy.

8. Serve warm.

233.Creamy-Cheesy Wontons

Prep time: 5 minutes | Cook time: 6 minutes | Serves 4

2 ounces (57 g) cream cheese, softened
1 tablespoon sugar
16 square wonton wrappers
Cooking spray

1. Spritz the air fry basket with cooking spray.

2. In a mixing bowl, stir together the sugar and cream cheese until well mixed. Prepare a small bowl of water alongside.

3. On a clean work surface, lay the wonton wrappers. Scoop ¼ teaspoon of cream cheese in the center of each wonton wrapper. Dab the water over the wrapper edges. Fold each wonton wrapper diagonally in half over the filling to form a triangle.

4. Arrange the wontons in the basket. Spritz the wontons with cooking spray.

5. Place the basket on the air fry position.

6. Select Air Fry, set temperature to 350ºF (180ºC) and set time to 6 minutes. Flip the wontons halfway through the cooking time.

7. When cooking is complete, the wontons will be golden brown and crispy.

8. Divide the wontons among four plates. Let rest for 5 minutes before serving.

234.Golden Chicken Empanadas

Prep time: 25 minutes | Cook time: 12 minutes | Makes 12 empanadas

1 cup boneless, skinless rotisserie chicken breast meat, chopped finely
¼ cup salsa verde
$^2/_3$ cup shredded Cheddar cheese
1 teaspoon ground cumin
1 teaspoon ground black pepper
2 purchased refrigerated pie crusts, from a minimum 14.1-ounce (400 g) box

1 large egg

2 tablespoons water

Cooking spray

1.   Spritz the air fry basket with cooking spray. Set aside.

2.   Combine the chicken meat, Cheddar, salsa verde, cumin, and black pepper in a large bowl. Stir to mix well. Set aside.

3.   Unfold the pie crusts on a clean work surface, then use a large cookie cutter to cut out 3½-inch circles as much as possible.

4.   Roll the remaining crusts to a ball and flatten into a circle which has the same thickness of the original crust. Cut out more 3½-inch circles until you have 12 circles in total.

5.   Make the empanadas: Divide the chicken mixture in the middle of each circle, about 1½ tablespoons each. Dab the edges of the circle with water. Fold the circle in half over the filling to shape like a half-moon and press to seal, or you can press with a fork.

6.   Whisk the egg with water in a small bowl.

7.   Arrange the empanadas in the basket and spritz with cooking spray. Brush with whisked egg.

8.   Place the basket on the air fry position.

9.   Select Air Fry, set temperature to 350ºF (180ºC) and set time to 12 minutes. Flip the empanadas halfway through the cooking time.

10.   When cooking is complete, the empanadas will be golden and crispy.

11.   Serve immediately.

235..Fast Cheesy Bacon and Egg Wraps

Prep time: 15 minutes | Cook time: 10 minutes | Serves 3

3 corn tortillas

3 slices bacon, cut into strips

2 scrambled eggs

3 tablespoons salsa

1 cup grated Pepper Jack cheese

3 tablespoons cream cheese, divided

Cooking spray

1.   Spritz the air fry basket with cooking spray.

2.   Unfold the tortillas on a clean work surface, divide the bacon and eggs in the middle of the tortillas, then spread with scatter and salsa with cheeses. Fold the tortillas over.

3.   Arrange the tortillas in the basket.

4.   Place the basket on the air fry position.

5.   Select Air Fry, set temperature to 390ºF (199ºC) and set time to 10 minutes. Flip the tortillas halfway through the cooking time.

6.   When cooking is complete, the cheeses will be melted and the tortillas will be lightly browned.

7.   Serve immediately.

236.Beef and Seeds Burgers

Prep time: 15 minutes | Cook time: 10 minutes | Serves 4

1 teaspoon cumin seeds

1 teaspoon mustard seeds

1 teaspoon coriander seeds

1 teaspoon dried minced garlic

1 teaspoon dried red pepper flakes

1 teaspoon kosher salt

2 teaspoons ground black pepper

1 pound (454 g) 85% lean ground beef

2 tablespoons Worcestershire sauce

4 hamburger buns

Mayonnaise, for serving

Cooking spray

1.   Spritz the air fry basket with cooking spray.

2.   Put the garlic, seeds, salt, red pepper flakes, and ground black pepper in a food processor. Pulse to coarsely ground the mixture.

3.   Put the ground beef in a large bowl. Pour in the seed mixture and drizzle with Worcestershire sauce. Stir to mix well.

4.   Divide the mixture into four parts and shape each part into a ball, then bash each ball into a patty. Arrange the patties in the basket.

5.   Place the basket on the air fry position.

6.   Select Air Fry, set temperature to 350ºF (180ºC) and set time to 10 minutes. Flip the patties with tongs halfway through the cooking time.

7.   When cooked, the patties will be well browned.

8.   Assemble the buns with the patties, then drizzle the mayo over the patties to make the burgers. Serve immediately.

237.Thai Pork Burgers

Prep time: 10 minutes | Cook time: 14 minutes | Makes 6 sliders

1 pound (454 g) ground pork

1 tablespoon Thai curry paste

1½ tablespoons fish sauce

¼ cup thinly sliced scallions, white and green parts

2 tablespoons minced peeled fresh ginger

1 tablespoon light brown sugar

1 teaspoon ground black pepper

6 slider buns, split open lengthwise, warmed

Cooking spray

1.   Spritz the air fry basket with cooking spray.

2.   Combine all the ingredients, except for the buns in a large bowl. Stir to mix well.

3.   Divide and shape the mixture into six balls, then bash the balls into six 3-inch-diameter patties.

4.   Arrange the patties in the basket and spritz with cooking spray.

5.   Place the basket on the air fry position.

6.   Select Air Fry, set temperature to 375ºF (190ºC) and set time to 14 minutes. Flip the patties halfway through the cooking time.

7.   When cooked, the patties should be well browned.

8.   Assemble the buns with patties to make the sliders and serve immediately.

CHAPTER 12 HOLIDAY SPECIALS

238.Crispy Arancini

Prep time: 5 minutes | Cook time: 30 minutes | Makes 10 arancini

$^2/_3$ cup raw white Arborio rice
2 teaspoons butter
½ teaspoon salt
$1^1/_3$ cups water
2 large eggs, well beaten
1¼ cups seasoned Italian-style dried bread crumbs
10 ¾-inch semi-firm Mozzarella cubes
Cooking spray

1.   Pour the rice, salt, butter, and water in a pot. Stir to mix well and bring a boil over medium-high heat. Keep stirring.
2.   Reduce the heat to low and cover the pot. Simmer for 20 minutes or until the rice is tender.
3.   Turn off the heat and let sit, covered, for 10 minutes, then open the lid and fluffy the rice with a fork. Allow to cool for 10 more minutes.
4.   Pour the beaten eggs in a bowl, then pour the bread crumbs in a separate bowl.
5.   Scoop 2 tablespoons of the cooked rice up and form it into a ball, then press the Mozzarella into the ball and wrap.
6.   Dredge the ball in the eggs first, then shake the excess off the dunk the ball in the bread crumbs. Roll to coat evenly. Repeat to make 10 balls in total with remaining rice.
7.   Transfer the balls in the air fry basket and spritz with cooking spray.
8.   Place the basket on the air fry position.
9.   Select Air Fry, set temperature to 375ºF (190ºC) and set time to 10 minutes.
10.   When cooking is complete, the balls should be lightly browned and crispy.
11.   Remove the balls from the air fryer grill and allow to cool before serving.

239..Fast Banana Cake

Prep time: 25 minutes | Cook time: 20 minutes | Serves 8

1 cup plus 1 tablespoon all-purpose flour
¼ teaspoon baking soda
¾ teaspoon baking powder
¼ teaspoon salt
9½ tablespoons granulated white sugar
5 tablespoons butter, at room temperature
2½ small ripe bananas, peeled
2 large eggs
5 tablespoons buttermilk
1 teaspoon vanilla extract
Cooking spray

1.   Spritz a baking pan with cooking spray.
2.   Combine the flour, baking powder, salt, and baking soda in a large bowl. Stir to mix well.
3.   Beat the sugar and butter in a separate bowl with a hand mixer on medium speed for 3 minutes.
4.   Beat in the bananas, eggs, vanilla, and buttermilk extract into the sugar and butter mix with a hand mixer.
5.   Pour in the flour mixture and whip with hand mixer until sanity and smooth.
6.   Scrape the batter into the pan and level the batter with a spatula.
7.   Place the pan on the bake position.
8.   Select Bake, set temperature to 325ºF (163ºC) and set time to 20 minutes.
9.   After 15 minutes, remove the pan from the air fryer grill. Check the doneness. Return the pan to the air fryer grill and continue cooking.
10.   When done, a toothpick inserted in the center should come out clean.
11.   Invert the cake on a cooling rack and allow to cool for 15 minutes before slicing to serve.

240.Sausage Rolls

Prep time: 10 minutes | Cook time: 8 minutes | Makes 16 rolls

1 can refrigerated crescent roll dough
1 small package mini smoked sausages, patted dry
2 tablespoons melted butter
2 teaspoons sesame seeds
1 teaspoon onion powder

1.   Place the crescent roll dough on a clean work surface and separate into 8 pieces. Cut each piece in half and you will have 16 triangles.

2.	Make the pigs in the blanket: Arrange each sausage on each dough triangle, then roll the sausages up.

3.	Brush the pigs with melted butter and place of the pigs in the blanket in the air fry basket. Sprinkle with sesame seeds and onion powder.

4.	Place the basket on the bake position.

5.	Select Bake, set temperature to 330ºF (166ºC) and set time to 8 minutes. Flip the pigs halfway through the cooking time.

6.	When cooking is complete, the pigs should be fluffy and golden brown.

7.	Serve immediately.

241.Blistered Cherry Tomatoes

Prep time: 5 minutes | Cook time: 10 minutes | Serves 4 to 6

2 pounds (907 g) cherry tomatoes
2 tablespoons olive oil
2 teaspoons balsamic vinegar
½ teaspoon salt
½ teaspoon ground black pepper

1.	Toss the cherry tomatoes with olive oil in a large bowl to coat well. Pour the tomatoes in a baking pan.

2.	Slide the pan into the air fryer grill.

3.	Select Air Fry, set temperature to 400ºF (205ºC) and set time to 10 minutes. Stir the tomatoes halfway through the cooking time.

4.	When cooking is complete, the tomatoes will be blistered and lightly wilted.

5.	Transfer the blistered tomatoes to a large bowl and toss with balsamic vinegar, salt, and black pepper before serving.

242.Fast Golden Nuggets

Prep time: 15 minutes | Cook time: 4 minutes | Makes 20 nuggets

 1 cup all-purpose flour, plus more for dusting
1 teaspoon baking powder
½ teaspoon butter, at room temperature, plus more for brushing
¼ teaspoon salt
¼ cup water
⅛ teaspoon onion powder
¼ teaspoon garlic powder
⅛ teaspoon seasoning salt

Cooking spray

1.	Line the air fry basket with parchment paper.

2.	Mix the flour, butter, salt, and baking powder in a large bowl. Stir to mix well. Gradually whisk in the water until a sanity dough forms.

3.	Put the dough on a lightly floured work surface, then roll it out into a ½-inch thick rectangle with a rolling pin.

4.	Cut the dough into about twenty 1- or 2-inch squares, then arrange the squares in a single layer in the air fry basket. Spritz with cooking spray.

5.	Combine garlic powder, onion powder, and seasoning salt in a small bowl. Stir to mix well, then sprinkle the squares with the powder mixture.

6.	Place the basket on the air fry position.

7.	Select Air Fry, set temperature to 370ºF (188ºC) and set time to 4 minutes. Flip the squares halfway through the cooking time.

8.	When cooked, the dough squares should be golden brown.

9.	Remove the golden nuggets from the air fryer grill and brush with more butter immediately. Serve warm.

243..Golden Kale Salad Sushi Rolls

Prep time: 10 minutes | Cook time: 10 minutes | Serves 12

Kale Salad:
1½ cups chopped kale
1 tablespoon sesame seeds
¾ teaspoon soy sauce
¾ teaspoon toasted sesame oil
½ teaspoon rice vinegar
¼ teaspoon ginger
⅛ teaspoon garlic powder

Sushi Rolls:
3 sheets sushi nori
1 batch cauliflower rice
½ avocado, sliced

Sriracha Mayonnaise:
¼ cup Sriracha sauce
¼ cup vegan mayonnaise

Coating:
½ cup panko bread crumbs

1.	In a medium bowl, toss all the ingredients for the salad together until well coated and set aside.

2.	Place a sheet of nori on a clean work surface and spread the cauliflower rice in an even layer on the nori. Scoop 2 to 3 tablespoon of kale salad on the rice and spread over. Place 1 or 2 avocado slices on top. Roll up the sushi, pressing gently to get a nice, tight roll. Repeat to make the remaining 2 rolls.

3.	In a bowl, stir together the mayonnaise and Sriracha sauce until smooth. Add bread crumbs to a separate bowl.

4.	Dredge the sushi rolls in Sriracha Mayonnaise, then roll in bread crumbs till well coated.

5.	Place the coated sushi rolls in the air fry basket.

6.	Place the basket on the air fry position.

7.	Select Air Fry, set temperature to 390ºF (199ºC) and set time to 10 minutes. Flip the sushi rolls halfway through the cooking time.

8.	When cooking is complete, the sushi rolls will be golden brown and crispy. .

9.	Transfer to a platter and rest for 5 minutes before slicing each roll into 8 pieces. Serve warm.

244.Golden Chocolate and Coconut Macaroons

Prep time: 10 minutes | Cook time: 8 minutes |Makes 24 macaroons

3 large egg whites, at room temperature
¼ teaspoon salt
¾ cup granulated white sugar
4½ tablespoons unsweetened cocoa powder
2¼ cups unsweetened shredded coconut

1.	Line the air fry basket with parchment paper.

2.	Whisk the egg whites with salt in a large bowl with a hand mixer on high speed until stiff peaks form.

3.	Whisk in the sugar with the hand mixer on high speed until the mixture is thick. Mix in the cocoa powder and coconut.

4.	Scoop 2 tablespoons of the mixture and shape the mixture in a ball. Repeat with remaining mixture to make 24 balls in total.

5.	Arrange the balls in a single layer in the air fry basket and leave a little space between each two balls.

6.	Place the basket on the air fry position.

7.	Select Air Fry, set temperature to 375ºF (190ºC) and set time to 8 minutes.

8.	When cooking is complete, the balls should be golden brown.

9.	Serve immediately.

245.Milk-Butter Pecan Tart

Prep time: 2 hours 25 minutes | Cook time: 26 minutes | Serves 8
Tart Crust:
¼ cup firmly packed brown sugar
$1/_3$ cup butter, softened
1 cup all-purpose flour
¼ teaspoon kosher salt
Filling:
¼ cup whole milk
4 tablespoons butter, diced
½ cup packed brown sugar
¼ cup pure maple syrup
1½ cups finely chopped pecans
¼ teaspoon pure vanilla extract
¼ teaspoon sea salt

1.	Line a baking pan with aluminum foil, then spritz the pan with cooking spray.

2.	Stir the brown sugar and butter in a bowl with a hand mixer until puffed, then add the flour and salt and stir until crumbled.

3.	Pour the mixture in the prepared baking pan and tilt the pan to coat the bottom evenly.

4.	Place the pan on the bake position.Place the pan on the bake position.

5.	Select Bake, set temperature to 350ºF (180ºC) and set time to 13 minutes.

6.	When done, the crust will be golden brown.

7.	Meanwhile, pour the milk, butter, sugar, and maple syrup in a saucepan. Stir to mix well. Bring to a simmer, then cook for 1 more minute. Stir constantly.

8.	Turn off the heat and mix the pecans and vanilla into the filling mixture.

9.	Pour the filling mixture over the golden crust and spread with a spatula to coat the crust evenly.

10.	Place the pan on the bake position.

11. Select Bake and set time to 12 minutes. When cooked, the filling mixture should be set and frothy.

12. Remove the baking pan from the air fryer grill and sprinkle with salt. Allow to sit for 10 minutes or until cooled.

13. Transfer the pan to the refrigerator to chill for at least 2 hours, then remove the aluminum foil and slice to serve.

246.Cheese Bread (Pão de Queijo)

Prep time: 37 minutes | Cook time: 12 minutes | Makes 12 balls

2 tablespoons butter, plus more for greasing
½ cup milk
1½ cups tapioca flour
½ teaspoon salt
1 large egg
$^2/_3$ cup finely grated aged Asiago cheese

1. Put the butter in a saucepan and pour in the milk, heat over medium heat until the liquid boils. Keep stirring.

2. Turn off the heat and mix in the salt and tapioca flour to form a soft dough. Transfer the dough in a large bowl, then wrap the bowl in plastic and let sit for 15 minutes.

3. Break the egg in the bowl of dough and whisk with a hand mixer for 2 minutes or until a sanity dough forms. Fold the cheese in the dough. Cover the bowl in plastic again and let sit for 10 more minutes.

4. Grease a baking pan with butter.

5. Scoop 2 tablespoons of the dough into the baking pan. Repeat with the remaining dough to make dough 12 balls. Keep a little distance between each two balls.

6. Flip the balls halfway through the cooking time.

7. Select Bake, set temperature to 375ºF (190ºC) and set time to 12 minutes.

8. When cooking is complete, the balls should be golden brown and fluffy.

9. Remove the balls from the air fryer grill and allow to cool for 5 minutes before serving.

247.Golden Garlicky Olive Stromboli

Prep time: 25 minutes | Cook time: 25 minutes | Serves 8

4 large cloves garlic, unpeeled
3 tablespoons grated Parmesan cheese
½ cup packed fresh basil leaves
½ cup marinated, pitted green and black olives
¼ teaspoon crushed red pepper
½ pound (227 g) pizza dough, at room temperature
4 ounces (113 g) sliced provolone cheese (about 8 slices)
Cooking spray

1. Spritz the air fry basket with cooking spray. Put the unpeeled garlic in the air fry basket.

2. Place the basket on the air fry position.

3. Select Air Fry, set temperature to 370ºF (188ºC) and set time to 10 minutes.

4. When cooked, the garlic will be softened completely. Remove from the air fryer grill and allow to cool until you can handle.

5. Peel the garlic and place into a food processor with 2 tablespoons of basil, crushed red pepper, Parmesan, and olives. Pulse to mix well. Set aside.

6. Arrange the pizza dough on a clean work surface, then roll it out with a rolling pin into a rectangle. Cut the rectangle in half.

7. Sprinkle half of the garlic mixture over each rectangle half, and leave ½-inch edges uncover. Top them with the provolone cheese.

8. Brush one long side of each rectangle half with water, then roll them up. Spritz the air fry basket with cooking spray. Transfer the rolls to the air fry basket. Spritz with cooking spray and scatter with remaining Parmesan.

9. Place the basket on the air fry position.

10. Select Air Fry and set time to 15 minutes. Flip the rolls halfway through the cooking time. When done, the rolls should be golden brown.

11. Remove the rolls from the air fryer grill and allow to cool for a few minutes before serving.

248.Simple Chocolate Buttermilk Cake

Prep time: 20 minutes | Cook time: 20 minutes | Serves 8

1 cup all-purpose flour
$^2/_3$ cup granulated white sugar
¼ cup unsweetened cocoa powder

¾ teaspoon baking soda

¼ teaspoon salt

$^2/_3$ cup buttermilk

2 tablespoons plus 2 teaspoons vegetable oil

1 teaspoon vanilla extract

Cooking spray

1.	Spritz a baking pan with cooking spray.

2.	Combine the flour, cocoa powder, sugar, salt, and baking soda in a large bowl. Stir to mix well.

3.	Mix in the buttermilk, vegetable oil, and vanilla. Keep stirring until it forms a grainy and thick dough.

4.	Scrape the chocolate batter from the bowl and transfer to the pan, level the batter in an even layer with a spatula.

5.	Place the pan on the bake position.

6.	Select Bake, set temperature to 325ºF (163ºC) and set time to 20 minutes.

7.	After 15 minutes, remove the pan from the air fryer grill. Check the doneness. Return the pan to the air fryer grill and continue cooking.

8.	When done, a toothpick inserted in the center should come out clean.

9.	Invert the cake on a cooling rack and allow to cool for 15 minutes before slicing to serve.

249.Chocolate-Glazed Custard Donut Holes

Prep time: 1 hour 50 minutes | Cook time: 4 minutes | Makes 24 donut holes
Dough:

1½ cups bread flour

2 egg yolks

1 teaspoon active dry yeast

½ cup warm milk

½ teaspoon pure vanilla extract

2 tablespoons butter, melted

1 tablespoon sugar

¼ teaspoon salt

Cooking spray

Custard Filling:

1 (3.4-ounce / 96-g) box French vanilla instant pudding mix

¼ cup heavy cream

¾ cup whole milk

Chocolate Glaze:

$^1/_3$ cup heavy cream

1 cup chocolate chips

Special Equipment:

A pastry bag with a long tip

1.	Combine the ingredients for the dough in a food processor, then pulse until a satiny dough ball forms.

2.	Transfer the dough on a lightly floured work surface, then knead for 2 minutes by hand and shape the dough back to a ball.

3.	Spritz a large bowl with cooking spray, then transfer the dough ball into the bowl. Wrap the bowl in plastic and let it rise for 1½ hours or until it doubled in size.

4.	Transfer the risen dough on a floured work surface, then shape it into a 24-inch long log. Cut the log into 24 parts and shape each part into a ball.

5.	Transfer the balls on two baking sheets and let sit to rise for 30 more minutes.

6.	Spritz the balls with cooking spray.

7.	Place the baking sheets on the bake position.

8.	Select Bake, set temperature to 400ºF (205ºC) and set time to 4 minutes. Flip the balls halfway through the cooking time.

9.	When cooked, the balls should be golden brown.

10.	Meanwhile, combine the ingredients for the filling in a large bowl and whisk for 2 minutes with a hand mixer until well combined.

11.	Pour the heavy cream in a saucepan, then bring to a boil. Put the chocolate chips in a small bowl and pour in the boiled heavy cream immediately. Mix until the chocolate chips are melted and the mixture is smooth.

12.	Transfer the baked donut holes to a large plate, then pierce a hole into each donut hole and lightly hollow them.

13.	Pour the filling in a pastry bag with a long tip and gently squeeze the filling into the donut holes. Then top the donut holes with chocolate glaze.

14.	Allow to sit for 10 minutes, then serve.

250.Easy Butter Cake

Prep time: 25 minutes | Cook time: 20 minutes | Serves 8

1 cup all-purpose flour

1¼ teaspoons baking powder

¼ teaspoon salt

½ cup plus 1½ tablespoons granulated white sugar

9½ tablespoons butter, at room temperature

2 large eggs

1 large egg yolk

2½ tablespoons milk

1 teaspoon vanilla extract

Cooking spray

1. Spritz a baking pan with cooking spray.

2. Combine the flour, salt, and baking powder in a large bowl. Stir to mix well.

3. Whip the sugar and butter in a separate bowl with a hand mixer on medium speed for 3 minutes.

4. Whip the egg yolk, eggs, milk, and vanilla extract into the sugar and butter mix with a hand mixer.

5. Pour in the flour mixture and whip with hand mixer until sanity and smooth.

6. Scrape the batter into the baking pan and level the batter with a spatula.

7. Place the pan on the bake position.

8. Select Bake, set temperature to 325ºF (163ºC) and set time to 20 minutes.

9. After 15 minutes, remove the pan from the air fryer grill. Check the doneness. Return the pan to the air fryer grill and continue cooking.

10. When done, a toothpick inserted in the center should come out clean.

11. Invert the cake on a cooling rack and allow to cool for 15 minutes before slicing to serve.

251.Golden Jewish Blintzes

Prep time: 5 minutes | Cook time: 10 minutes | Makes 8 blintzes

2 (7½-ounce / 213-g) packages farmer cheese, mashed

¼ cup cream cheese

¼ teaspoon vanilla extract

¼ cup granulated white sugar

8 egg roll wrappers

4 tablespoons butter, melted

1. Combine the cream cheese, farmer cheese, sugar, and vanilla extract in a bowl. Stir to mix well.

2. Unfold the egg roll wrappers on a clean work surface, spread ¼ cup of the filling at the edge of each wrapper and leave a ½-inch edge uncovering.

3. Wet the edges of the wrappers with water and fold the uncovered edge over the filling. Fold the left and right sides in the center, then tuck the edge under the filling and fold to wrap the filling.

4. Brush the wrappers with melted butter, then arrange the wrappers in a single layer in the air fry basket, seam side down. Leave a little space between each two wrappers.

5. Place the basket on the air fry position.

6. Select Air Fry, set temperature to 375ºF (190ºC) and set time to 10 minutes.

7. When cooking is complete, the wrappers will be golden brown.

8. Serve immediately.

252..Fast Teriyaki Shrimp Skewers

Prep time: 10 minutes | Cook time: 6 minutes | Makes 12 skewered shrimp

1½ tablespoons mirin

1½ teaspoons ginger juice

1½ tablespoons soy sauce

12 large shrimp (about 20 shrimps per pound), peeled and deveined

1 large egg

¾ cup panko bread crumbs

Cooking spray

1. Combine the mirin, soy sauce, and ginger juice in a large bowl. Stir to mix well.

2. Dunk the shrimp in the bowl of mirin mixture, then wrap the bowl in plastic and refrigerate for 1 hour to marinate.

3. Spritz the air fry basket with cooking spray.

4. Run twelve 4-inch skewers through each shrimp.

5. Whisk the egg in the bowl of marinade to combine well. Pour the bread crumbs on a plate.

6. Dredge the shrimp skewers in the egg mixture, then shake the excess off and roll over the bread crumbs to coat well.

7. Arrange the shrimp skewers in the air fry basket and spritz with cooking spray.

8. Place the basket on the air fry position.

9. Select Air Fry, set temperature to 400ºF (205ºC) and set time to 6 minutes. Flip the shrimp skewers halfway through the cooking time.

10. When done, the shrimp will be opaque and firm.

11.   Serve immediately.

253..Cream Glazed Cinnamon Rolls

Prep time: 2 hours 15 minutes | Cook time: 5 minutes | Serves 8

1 pound (454 g) frozen bread dough, thawed
2 tablespoons melted butter
1½ tablespoons cinnamon
¾ cup brown sugar
Cooking spray

Cream Glaze:

4 ounces (113 g) softened cream cheese
½ teaspoon vanilla extract
2 tablespoons melted butter
1¼ cups powdered erythritol

1.   Place the bread dough on a clean work surface, then roll the dough out into a rectangle with a rolling pin.
2.   Brush the top of the dough with melted butter and leave 1-inch edges uncovered.
3.   Combine the cinnamon and sugar in a small bowl, then sprinkle the dough with the cinnamon mixture.
4.   Roll the dough over tightly, then cut the dough log into 8 portions. Wrap the portions in plastic, better separately, and let sit to rise for 1 or 2 hours.
5.   Meanwhile, combine the ingredients for the glaze in a separate small bowl. Stir to mix well.
6.   Spritz the air fry basket with cooking spray. Transfer the risen rolls to the air fry basket.
7.   Place the basket on the air fry position.
8.   Select Air Fry, set temperature to 350ºF (180ºC) and set time to 5 minutes. Flip the rolls halfway through the cooking time.
9.   When cooking is complete, the rolls will be golden brown.
10.   Serve the rolls with the glaze.

CHAPTER 13 FAST AND EASY EVERYDAY FAVORITES

254..Fast Traditional Latkes

Prep time: 15 minutes | Cook time: 10 minutes | | Makes 4 latkes

1 egg

2 tablespoons all-purpose flour

2 medium potatoes, peeled and shredded, rinsed and drained

¼ teaspoon granulated garlic

½ teaspoon salt

Cooking spray

1.   Spritz the air fry basket with cooking spray.

2.   Whisk together the egg, flour, potatoes, garlic, and salt in a large bowl. Stir to mix well.

3.   Divide the mixture into four parts, then flatten them into four circles. Arrange the circles onto the air fry basket and spritz with cooking spray.

4.   Place the basket on the air fry position.

5.   Select Air Fry, set temperature to 380ºF (193ºC) and set time to 10 minutes. Flip the latkes halfway through.

6.   When cooked, the latkes will be golden brown and crispy. Remove the basket from the air fryer grill.

7.   Serve immediately.

255.Simple Garlicky-Cheesy Shrimps

Prep time: 10 minutes | Cook time: 8 minutes | Serves 4 to 6

²/₃ cup grated Parmesan cheese

4 minced garlic cloves

1 teaspoon onion powder

½ teaspoon oregano

1 teaspoon basil

1 teaspoon ground black pepper

2 tablespoons olive oil

2 pounds (907 g) cooked large shrimps, peeled and deveined

Lemon wedges, for topping

Cooking spray

1.   Spritz the air fry basket with cooking spray.

2.   Combine all the ingredients, except for the shrimps, in a large bowl. Stir to mix well.

3.   Dunk the shrimps in the mixture and toss to coat well. Shake the excess off. Arrange the shrimps in the air fry basket.

4.   Place the basket on the air fry position.

5.   Select Air Fry, set temperature to 350ºF (180ºC) and set time to 8 minutes. Flip the shrimps halfway through the cooking time.

6.   When cooking is complete, the shrimps should be opaque. Remove the pan from the air fryer grill.

7.   Transfer the cooked shrimps on a large plate and squeeze the lemon wedges over before serving.

256.Fast Baked Cherry Tomatoes

Prep time: 5 minutes | Cook time: 5 minutes | Serves 2

2 cups cherry tomatoes

1 clove garlic, thinly sliced

1 teaspoon olive oil

⅛ teaspoon kosher salt

1 tablespoon freshly chopped basil, for topping

Cooking spray

1.   Spritz a baking pan with cooking spray and set aside.

2.   In a large bowl, toss together the cherry tomatoes, sliced garlic, olive oil, and kosher salt. Spread the mixture in an even layer in the prepared pan.

3.   Place the pan on the bake position.

4.   Select Bake, set temperature to 360ºF (182ºC) and set time to 5 minutes.

5.   When cooking is complete, the tomatoes should be the soft and wilted.

6.   Transfer to a bowl and rest for 5 minutes. Top with the chopped basil and serve warm.

257.Easy Air-Fried Edamame

Prep time: 5 minutes | Cook time: 7 minutes | Serves 6

1½ pounds (680 g) unshelled edamame

2 tablespoons olive oil

1 teaspoon sea salt

1.	Place the edamame in a large bowl, then drizzle with olive oil. Toss to coat well. Transfer the edamame to the air fry basket.

2.	Place the basket on the air fry position.

3.	Select Air Fry, set temperature to 400ºF (205ºC) and set time to 7 minutes. Stir the edamame at least three times during cooking.

4.	When done, the edamame will be tender and warmed through.

5.	Transfer the cooked edamame onto a plate and sprinkle with salt. Toss to combine well and set aside for 3 minutes to infuse before serving.

258..Easy Spicy Old Bay Shrimp

Prep time: 10 minutes | Cook time: 10 minutes | Makes 2 cups

½ teaspoon Old Bay Seasoning
1 teaspoon ground cayenne pepper
½ teaspoon paprika
1 tablespoon olive oil
⅛ teaspoon salt
½ pound (227 g) shrimps, peeled and deveined
Juice of half a lemon

1.	Combine the Old Bay Seasoning, olive oil, salt, paprika, and cayenne pepper in a large bowl, then add the shrimps and toss to coat well.

2.	Put the shrimps in the air fry basket.

3.	Place the basket on the air fry position.

4.	Select Air Fry, set temperature to 390ºF (199ºC) and set time to 10 minutes. Flip the shrimps halfway through the cooking time.

5.	When cooking is complete, the shrimps should be opaque. Remove from the air fryer grill.

6.	Serve the shrimps with lemon juice on top.

259.Fast Corn on the Cob

Prep time: 10 minutes | Cook time: 10 minutes | Serves 4

2 tablespoons mayonnaise
2 teaspoons minced garlic
½ teaspoon sea salt
1 cup panko bread crumbs
4 (4-inch length) ears corn on the cob, husk and silk removed
Cooking spray

1.	Spritz the air fry basket with cooking spray.

2.	Combine the garlic, mayonnaise, and salt in a bowl. Stir to mix well. Pour the panko on a plate.

3.	Brush the corn on the cob with mayonnaise mixture, then roll the cob in the bread crumbs and press to coat well.

4.	Transfer the corn on the cob in the air fry basket and spritz with cooking spray.

5.	Place the basket on the air fry position.

6.	Select Air Fry, set temperature to 400ºF (205ºC) and set time to 10 minutes. Flip the corn on the cob at least three times during the cooking.

7.	When cooked, the corn kernels on the cob should be almost browned. Remove the basket from the air fryer grill.

8.	Serve immediately.

260.Golden Worcestershire Poutine

Prep time: 15 minutes | Cook time: 33 minutes | Serves 2

2 russet potatoes, scrubbed and cut into ½-inch sticks
2 teaspoons vegetable oil
2 tablespoons butter
¼ onion, minced
¼ teaspoon dried thyme
1 clove garlic, smashed
3 tablespoons all-purpose flour
1 teaspoon tomato paste
1½ cups beef stock
2 teaspoons Worcestershire sauce
Salt and freshly ground black pepper, to taste
$^2/_3$ cup chopped string cheese

1.	Bring a pot of water to a boil, then put in the potato sticks and blanch for 4 minutes.

2.	Drain the potato sticks and rinse under running cold water, then pat dry with paper towels.

3.	Transfer the sticks in a large bowl and drizzle with vegetable oil. Toss to coat well. Place the potato sticks in the air fry basket.

4.	Place the basket on the air fry position.

5.	Select Air Fry, set temperature to 400ºF (205ºC) and set time to 25 minutes. Stir the potato sticks at least three times during cooking.

6.	Meanwhile, make the gravy: Heat the butter in a saucepan over medium heat until melted.

7.	Add the onion, garlic, and thyme and sauté for 5 minutes or until the onion is translucent.

8. Add the flour and sauté for an additional 2 minutes. Pour in the tomato paste and beef stock and cook for 1 more minute or until lightly thickened.
9. Drizzle the gravy with Worcestershire sauce and sprinkle with salt and ground black pepper. Reduce the heat to low to keep the gravy warm until ready to serve.
10. When done, the sticks should be golden brown. Remove the basket from the air fryer grill. Transfer the fried potato sticks onto a plate, then sprinkle with salt and ground black pepper. Scatter with string cheese and pour the gravy over. Serve warm.

261.Sugary Glazed Apple Fritters

Prep time: 10 minutes | Cook time: 8 minutes | Makes 15 fritters
Apple Fritters:
2 firm apples, peeled, cored, and diced
½ teaspoon cinnamon
Juice of 1 lemon
1 cup all-purpose flour
1½ teaspoons baking powder
½ teaspoon kosher salt
2 eggs
¼ cup milk
2 tablespoons unsalted butter, melted
2 tablespoons granulated sugar
Cooking spray
Glaze:
½ teaspoon vanilla extract
1¼ cups powdered sugar, sifted
¼ cup water
1. Line the air fry basket with parchment paper.
2. Combine the apples with lemon juice and cinnamon in a small bowl. Toss to coat well.
3. Combine the flour, baking powder, and salt in a large bowl. Stir to mix well.
4. Whisk the egg, butter, milk, and sugar in a medium bowl. Stir to mix well.
5. Make a well in the center of the flour mixture, then pour the egg mixture into the well and stir to mix well. Mix in the apple until a dough forms.
6. Use an ice cream scoop to scoop 15 balls from the dough onto the pan. Spritz with cooking spray.

7. Place the basket on the air fry position.
8. Select Air Fry, set temperature to 360ºF (182ºC) and set time to 8 minutes. Flip the apple fritters halfway through the cooking time.
9. Meanwhile, combine the ingredients for the glaze in a separate small bowl. Stir to mix well.
10. When cooking is complete, the apple fritters will be golden brown. Serve the fritters with the glaze on top or use the glaze for dipping.

262.Chessy Jalapeño Cornbread

Prep time: 10 minutes | Cook time: 20 minutes | Serves 8
²/₃ cup cornmeal
¹/₃ cup all-purpose flour
¾ teaspoon baking powder
2 tablespoons buttery spread, melted
½ teaspoon kosher salt
1 tablespoon granulated sugar
¾ cup whole milk
1 large egg, beaten
1 jalapeño pepper, thinly sliced
¹/₃ cup shredded sharp Cheddar cheese
Cooking spray
1. Spritz a baking pan with cooking spray.
2. Combine all the ingredients in a large bowl. Stir to mix well. Pour the mixture in the baking pan.
3. Place the pan on the bake position.
4. Select Bake, set temperature to 300ºF (150ºC) and set time to 20 minutes.
5. When the cooking is complete, a toothpick inserted in the center of the bread should come out clean.
6. Remove the baking pan from the air fryer grill and allow the bread to cool for 5 minutes before slicing to serve.

263..Panko Salmon and Carrot Croquettes

Prep time: 15 minutes | Cook time: 10 minutes | Serves 6
2 egg whites
1 cup almond flour
1 cup panko bread crumbs
1 pound (454 g) chopped salmon fillet
²/₃ cup grated carrots
2 tablespoons minced garlic cloves
½ cup chopped onion

2 tablespoons chopped chives
Cooking spray

1. Spritz the air fry basket with cooking spray.
2. Whisk the egg whites in a bowl. Put the flour in a second bowl. Pour the bread crumbs in a third bowl. Set aside.
3. Combine the salmon, garlic, onion, carrots, and chives in a large bowl. Stir to mix well.
4. Form the mixture into balls with your hands. Dredge the balls into the flour, then egg, and then bread crumbs to coat well.
5. Arrange the salmon balls in the air fry basket and spritz with cooking spray.
6. Place the basket on the air fry position.
7. Select Air Fry, set temperature to 350ºF (180ºC) and set time to 10 minutes. Flip the salmon balls halfway through cooking.
8. When cooking is complete, the salmon balls will be crispy and browned. Remove the basket from the air fryer grill.
9. Serve immediately.

264..Spicy Chicken Wings

Prep time: 5 minutes | Cook time: 15 minutes | Makes 16 wings

16 chicken wings
3 tablespoons hot sauce
Cooking spray

10. Spritz the air fry basket with cooking spray.
11. Arrange the chicken wings in the air fry basket.
12. Place the basket on the air fry position.
13. Select Air Fry, set temperature to 360ºF (182ºC) and set time to 15 minutes. Flip the wings at lease three times during cooking.
14. When cooking is complete, the chicken wings will be well browned. Remove the pan from the air fryer grill.
15. Transfer the air fried wings to a plate and serve with hot sauce.

265.Air-Fried Lemony Shishito Peppers

Prep time: 5 minutes | Cook time: 5 minutes | Serves 4

½ pound (227 g) shishito peppers (about 24)
1 tablespoon olive oil
Coarse sea salt, to taste

Lemon wedges, for serving
Cooking spray

1. Spritz the air fry basket with cooking spray.
2. Toss the peppers with olive oil in a large bowl to coat well.
3. Arrange the peppers in the air fry basket.
4. Place the basket on the air fry position.
5. Select Air Fry, set temperature to 400ºF (205ºC) and set time to 5 minutes. Flip the peppers and sprinkle the peppers with salt halfway through the cooking time.
6. When cooked, the peppers should be blistered and lightly charred. Transfer the peppers onto a plate and squeeze the lemon wedges on top before serving.

266.Greek Spanakopita

Prep time: 10 minutes | Cook time: 8 minutes | Serves 6

½ (10-ounce / 284-g) package frozen spinach, thawed and squeezed dry
1 egg, lightly beaten
¼ cup pine nuts, toasted
¼ cup grated Parmesan cheese
¾ cup crumbled feta cheese
⅛ teaspoon ground nutmeg
½ teaspoon salt
Freshly ground black pepper, to taste
6 sheets phyllo dough
½ cup butter, melted

1. Combine all the ingredients, except for the phyllo dough and butter, in a large bowl. Whisk to combine well. Set aside.
2. Place a sheet of phyllo dough on a clean work surface. Brush with butter then top with another layer sheet of phyllo. Brush with butter, then cut the layered sheets into six 3-inch-wide strips.
3. Top each strip with 1 tablespoon of the spinach mixture, then fold the bottom left corner over the mixture towards the right strip edge to make a triangle. Keep folding triangles until each strip is folded over.
4. Brush the triangles with butter and repeat with remaining strips and phyllo dough.
5. Place the triangles in the baking pan.
6. Place the pan into the air fryer grill.

7. Select Air Fry, set temperature to 350ºF (180ºC) and set time to 8 minutes. Flip the triangles halfway through the cooking time.

8. When cooking is complete, the triangles should be golden brown. Remove the pan from the air fryer grill.

9. Serve immediately.

267.Crunchy Sweet Cinnamon Chickpeas

Prep time: 10 minutes | Cook time: 10 minutes | Serves 2

1 tablespoon cinnamon
1 tablespoon sugar
1 cup chickpeas, soaked in water overnight, rinsed and drained

1. Combine the cinnamon and sugar in a bowl. Stir to mix well.

2. Add the chickpeas to the bowl, then toss to coat well.

3. Pour the chickpeas in the air fry basket.

4. Place the basket on the air fry position.

5. Select Air Fry, set temperature to 390ºF (199ºC) and set time to 10 minutes. Stir the chickpeas three times during cooking.

6. When cooked, the chickpeas should be golden brown and crispy. Remove the basket from the air fryer grill.

7. Serve immediately.

268.Air-Fried Squash with Hazelnuts

Prep time: 10 minutes | Cook time: 23 minutes | Makes 3 cups

2 tablespoons whole hazelnuts
3 cups butternut squash, peeled, deseeded and cubed
¼ teaspoon kosher salt
¼ teaspoon freshly ground black pepper
2 teaspoons olive oil
Cooking spray

1. Spritz the air fry basket with cooking spray. Spread the hazelnuts in the basket.

2. Place the basket on the air fry position.

3. Select Air Fry, set temperature to 300ºF (150ºC) and set time to 3 minutes.

4. When done, the hazelnuts should be soft. Remove from the air fryer grill. Chopped the hazelnuts roughly and transfer to a small bowl. Set aside.

5. Put the butternut squash in a large bowl, then sprinkle with salt and pepper and drizzle with

olive oil. Toss to coat well. Transfer the squash to the lightly greased basket.

6. Place the basket on the air fry position.

7. Select Air Fry, set temperature to 360ºF (182ºC) and set time to 20 minutes. Flip the squash halfway through the cooking time.

8. When cooking is complete, the squash will be soft. Transfer the squash to a plate and sprinkle with the chopped hazelnuts before serving.

269.Crispy Citrus Avocado Wedge Fries

Prep time: 10 minutes | Cook time: 8 minutes | Makes 12 fries

1 cup all-purpose flour
3 tablespoons lime juice
¾ cup orange juice
1¼ cups plain dried bread crumbs
1 cup yellow cornmeal
1½ tablespoons chile powder
2 large Hass avocados, peeled, pitted, and cut into wedges
Coarse sea salt, to taste
Cooking spray

1. Spritz the air fry basket with cooking spray.

2. Pour the flour in a bowl. Mix the lime juice with orange juice in a second bowl. Combine the cornmeal, bread crumbs, and chile powder in a third bowl.

3. Dip the avocado wedges in the bowl of flour to coat well, then dredge the wedges into the bowl of juice mixture, and then dunk the wedges in the bread crumbs mixture. Shake the excess off.

4. Arrange the coated avocado wedges in a single layer in the air fry basket. Spritz with cooking spray.

5. Place the basket on the air fry position.

6. Select Air Fry, set temperature to 400ºF (205ºC) and set time to 8 minutes. Stir the avocado wedges and sprinkle with salt halfway through the cooking time.

7. When cooking is complete, the avocado wedges should be tender and crispy.

8. Serve immediately.

270.Lemony-Cheesy Pears

Prep time: 10 minutes | Cook time: 8 minutes | Serves 4

2 large Bartlett pears, peeled, cut in half, cored
3 tablespoons melted butter

½ teaspoon ground ginger

¼ teaspoon ground cardamom

3 tablespoons brown sugar

½ cup whole-milk ricotta cheese

1 teaspoon pure lemon extract

1 teaspoon pure almond extract

1 tablespoon honey, plus additional for drizzling

1. Toss the pears with ginger, butter, sugar, and cardamom in a large bowl. Toss to coat well. Arrange the pears in a baking pan, cut side down.

2. Place the pan into the air fryer grill.

3. Select Air Fry, set temperature to 375ºF (190ºC) and set time to 8 minutes.

4. After 5 minutes, remove the pan and flip the pears. Return the pan to the air fryer grill and continue cooking.

5. When cooking is complete, the pears should be soft and browned. Remove the pan from the air fryer grill.

6. In the meantime, combine the remaining ingredients in a separate bowl. Whip for 1 minute with a hand mixer until the mixture is puffed.

7. Divide the mixture into four bowls, then put the pears over the mixture and drizzle with more honey to serve.

271.Crunchy Salty Tortilla Chips

Prep time: 5 minutes | Cook time: 10 minutes | Serves 4

4 six-inch corn tortillas, cut in half and slice into thirds

1 tablespoon canola oil

¼ teaspoon kosher salt

Cooking spray

1. Spritz the air fry basket with cooking spray.

2. On a clean work surface, brush the tortilla chips with canola oil, then transfer the chips to the air fry basket.

3. Place the basket on the air fry position.

4. Select Air Fry, set temperature to 360ºF (182ºC) and set time to 10 minutes. Flip the chips and sprinkle with salt halfway through the cooking time.

5. When cooked, the chips will be crunchy and lightly browned. Transfer the chips to a plate lined with paper towels. Serve immediately.

272.Air-Fried Okra Chips

Prep time: 5 minutes | Cook time: 16 minutes | Serves 6

2 pounds (907 g) fresh okra pods, cut into 1-inch pieces

2 tablespoons canola oil

1 teaspoon coarse sea salt

1. Stir the salt and oil in a bowl to mix well. Add the okra and toss to coat well. Place the okra in the air fry basket.

2. Place the basket on the air fry position.

3. Select Air Fry, set temperature to 400ºF (205ºC) and set time to 16 minutes. Flip the okra at least three times during cooking.

4. When cooked, the okra should be lightly browned. Remove from the air fryer grill.

5. Serve immediately.

273.Parsnip Fries with Garlicky Yogurt

Prep time: 10 minutes | Cook time: 10 minutes | Serves 4

3 medium parsnips, peeled, cut into sticks

¼ teaspoon kosher salt

1 teaspoon olive oil

1 garlic clove, unpeeled

Cooking spray

Dip:

¼ cup plain Greek yogurt

⅛ teaspoon garlic powder

1 tablespoon sour cream

¼ teaspoon kosher salt

Freshly ground black pepper, to taste

1. Spritz the air fry basket with cooking spray.

2. Put the parsnip sticks in a large bowl, then sprinkle with salt and drizzle with olive oil.

3. Transfer the parsnip into the air fry basket and add the garlic.

4. Place the basket on the air fry position.

5. Select Air Fry, set temperature to 360ºF (182ºC) and set time to 10 minutes. Stir the parsnip halfway through the cooking time.

6. Meanwhile, peel the garlic and crush it. Combine the crushed garlic with the ingredients for the dip. Stir to mix well.

7. When cooked, the parsnip sticks should be crisp. Remove the parsnip fries from the air fryer grill and serve with the dipping sauce.

274.Golden Bacon Pinwheels

Prep time: 5 minutes | Cook time: 10 minutes | Makes 8 pinwheels

1 sheet puff pastry
2 tablespoons maple syrup
¼ cup brown sugar
8 slices bacon
Ground black pepper, to taste
Cooking spray

1.   Spritz the air fry basket with cooking spray.
2.   Roll the puff pastry into a 10-inch square with a rolling pin on a clean work surface, then cut the pastry into 8 strips.
3.   Brush the strips with maple syrup and sprinkle with sugar, leaving a 1-inch far end uncovered.
4.   Arrange each slice of bacon on each strip, leaving a ⅛-inch length of bacon hang over the end close to you. Sprinkle with black pepper.
5.   From the end close to you, roll the strips into pinwheels, then dab the uncovered end with water and seal the rolls.
6.   Arrange the pinwheels in the air fry basket and spritz with cooking spray.
7.   Place the basket on the air fry position.
8.   Select Air Fry, set temperature to 360ºF (182ºC) and set time to 10 minutes. Flip the pinwheels halfway through.
9.   When cooking is complete, the pinwheels should be golden brown. Remove the pan from the air fryer grill.
10.   Serve immediately.

275.Crispy and Beery Onion Rings

Prep time: 10 minutes | Cook time: 16 minutes | Serves 2 to 4

$^2/_3$ cup all-purpose flour
1 teaspoon paprika
½ teaspoon baking soda
1 teaspoon salt
½ teaspoon freshly ground black pepper
1 egg, beaten
¾ cup beer
1½ cups bread crumbs
1 tablespoons olive oil
1 large Vidalia onion, peeled and sliced into ½-inch rings
Cooking spray

1.   Spritz the air fry basket with cooking spray.
2.   Combine the flour, salt, baking soda, paprika, and ground black pepper in a bowl. Stir to mix well.
3.   Combine the egg and beer in a separate bowl. Stir to mix well.
4.   Make a well in the center of the flour mixture, then pour the egg mixture in the well. Stir to mix everything well.
5.   Pour the bread crumbs and olive oil in a shallow plate. Stir to mix well.
6.   Dredge the onion rings gently into the flour and egg mixture, then shake the excess off and put into the plate of bread crumbs. Flip to coat the both sides well. Arrange the onion rings in the air fry basket.
7.   Place the basket on the air fry position.
8.   Select Air Fry, set temperature to 360ºF (182ºC) and set time to 16 minutes. Flip the rings and put the bottom rings to the top halfway through.
9.   When cooked, the rings will be golden brown and crunchy. Remove the pan from the air fryer grill.
10.   Serve immediately.

276.Classic French Fries

Prep time: 5 minutes | Cook time: 25 minutes | Serves 2

2 russet potatoes, peeled and cut into ½-inch sticks
2 teaspoons olive oil
Salt, to taste
¼ cup ketchup, for serving

1.   Bring a pot of salted water to a boil. Put the potato sticks into the pot and blanch for 4 minutes.
2.   Rinse the potatoes under running cold water and pat dry with paper towels.
3.   Put the potato sticks in a large bowl and drizzle with olive oil. Toss to coat well.
4.   Transfer the potato sticks to the air fry basket.
5.   Place the basket on the air fry position.
6.   Select Air Fry, set temperature to 400ºF (205ºC) and set time to 25 minutes. Stir the potato sticks and sprinkle with salt halfway through.
7.   When cooked, the potato sticks will be crispy and golden brown. Remove the French fries from the air fryer grill and serve with ketchup.

CHAPTER 14 ROTISSERIE RECIPES

277.Lemony Rotisserie Lamb Leg

Prep time: 25 minutes | Cook time: 1 hour 30 minutes | Serves 4 to 6
3 pounds (1.4 kg) leg of lamb, boned in
Marinade:
1 tablespoon lemon zest (about 1 lemon)
3 tablespoons lemon juice (about 1½ lemons)
3 cloves garlic, minced
1 teaspoon onion powder
1 teaspoon fresh thyme
¼ cup fresh oregano
¼ cup olive oil
1 teaspoon ground black pepper
Herb Dressing:
1 tablespoon lemon juice (about ½ lemon)
¼ cup chopped fresh oregano
1 teaspoon fresh thyme
1 tablespoon olive oil
1 teaspoon sea salt
Ground black pepper, to taste
1.   Place lamb leg into a large resealable plastic bag. Combine the ingredients for the marinade in a small bowl. Stir to mix well.
2.   Pour the marinade over the lamb, making sure the meat is completely coated. Seal the bag and place in the refrigerator. Marinate for 4 to 6 hours before air fryer grilling.
3.   Remove the lamb leg from the marinade. Using the rotisserie spit, push through the lamb leg and attach the rotisserie forks.
4.   If desired, place aluminum foil onto the drip pan. (It makes for easier clean-up!)
5.   Place the prepared lamb leg with rotisserie spit into the air fryer grill.
6.   Select Toast, set temperature to 350ºF (180ºC), Rotate, and set time to 1 hour 30 minutes. Baste with marinade for every 30 minutes.
7.   Meanwhile, combine the ingredients for the herb dressing in a bowl. Stir to mix well.
8.   When cooking is complete, remove the lamb leg using the rotisserie lift and, using hot pads or gloves, carefully remove the lamb leg from the spit.
9.   Cover lightly with aluminum foil for 8 to 10 minutes.
10.   Carve the leg and arrange on a platter,. Drizzle with herb dressing. Serve immediately.

278.Roasted Pears

Here's a healthy roasted fruit recipe that'll make your mouth drool!
Prep and Cooking time: 60 minutes | Serves: 3
Ingredients to use:
3 semi-ripe pears
1/2 cup icing sugar
2 tbsp. butter
1 tbsp. ground cinnamon
3/4 cup white wine
Step-by-step Directions to Cook it:
1.   Mix all the ingredients, except for pears.
2.   Prick the pears with a fork and let it soak in the wine mixture for 15 minutes.
3.   Roast in the preheated PowerXL Air Fryer Grill for 20 minutes.
Nutritional value per serving:
Calories: 103kcal, Carbs: 27g, Protein: 1g, Fat: 4g

279.Chicken Breast with Veggies

No matter what time of the year it is, this classic chicken dish in dinner can never go wrong.
Prep and Cooking time: 50 minutes | Serves: 4
Ingredients to use:
4 deboned chicken breasts
1 tbsp. dried Italian herbs
Salt & pepper
1 tbsp. paprika
1 large carrot, chopped
1 large potato, chopped
Step-by-step Directions to Cook it:
1.   Preheat the PowerXL Air Fryer Grill to 150ºC or 300ºF.
2.   Mix all the seasonings and coat the chicken and veggies.
3.   Roast the chicken and veggies for 30 minutes.
Nutritional value per serving:
Calories: 140kcal, Protein: 22.3 g, Fat: 0.5 g.

280.Roasted Spaghetti Squash

Here's something healthy to munch on that won't take up a lot of time to make.
Prep and Cooking time: 30 minutes | Serves: 4
Ingredients to use:
1 ripe squash

Salt & pepper

Step-by-step Directions to Cook it:

1.   Preheat the PowerXL Air Fryer Grill to 150ºC or 300ºF.

2.   Prick the outside of the cleaned squash with a fork.

3.   Roast it for 10 minutes.

4.   Cut the roasted squash and scrape out the strands.

5.   Sprinkle salt and pepper and serve.

Nutritional value per serving:

Calories: 42kcal, Carbs: 3g, Protein: 1g, Fat: 0.5g,

281.Toasted Rotisserie Pork Shoulder

Prep time: 30 minutes | Cook time: 4 hours 30 minutes | Serves 6 to 8

1 (5-pound / 2.3-kg) boneless pork shoulder

1 tablespoon kosher salt

Rub:

2 teaspoons ground black peppercorns

2 teaspoons ground mustard seed

2 tablespoons light brown sugar

1 teaspoon onion powder

1 teaspoon garlic powder

1 teaspoon paprika

Mop:

1 cup bourbon

1 small onion, granulated

¼ cup corn syrup

¼ cup ketchup

2 tablespoons brown mustard

½ cup light brown sugar

1.   Combine the ingredients for the rub in a small bowl. Stir to mix well.

2.   Season pork shoulder all over with rub, wrap in plastic, and place in refrigerator for 12 to 15 hours.

3.   Remove roast from the fridge and let meat stand at room temperature for 30 to 45 minutes. Season with kosher salt.

4.   Whisk ingredients for mop in a medium bowl. Set aside until ready to use.

5.   Using the rotisserie spit, push through the pork should and attach the rotisserie forks.

6.   If desired, place aluminum foil onto the drip pan. (It makes for easier clean-up!)

7.   Place the prepared pork with rotisserie spit into the air fryer grill.

8.   Select Toast, set temperature to 450ºF (235ºC), Rotate, and set time to 30 minutes.

9.   After 30 minutes, reduce the temperature to 250ºF (121ºC) and roast for 4 more hours or until an meat thermometer inserted in the center of the pork reads at least 145 ºF (63 ºC).

10.   After the first hour of cooking, apply mop over the pork for every 20 minutes.

11.   When cooking is complete, remove the pork using the rotisserie lift and, using hot pads or gloves, carefully remove the pork tenderloin from the spit.

12.   Let stand for 10 minutes before slicing and serving.

282.Roasted Italian Sausage

Here's a quick and yummy meal prep recipe for the people who are always on the go.

Prep and Cooking time: 30 minutes | Serves: 4

Ingredients to use:

4 Italian sausage

1 large potato, chopped

2 ounces mushroom, chopped

1tbsp Italian herbs

1 tbsp. paprika

Salt

1 clove garlic

2 tbsp.。 olive oil

Step-by-step Directions to Cook it:

1.   Mix the seasonings and oil in a pan and coat the sausages and veggies.

2.   Roast in the PowerXL Air Fryer Grill for 20 minutes.

Nutritional value per serving:

Calories: 81kcal, Carbs: 60g, Protein: 4.7g, Fat: 7g

283.Slow Roasted Herb Chicken

If you want your chicken dinner to be both healthy and yummy, this recipe is here to pack the punch.

Prep and Cooking time: 60 minutes | Serves: 4

Ingredients to Use:

1 lb. whole chicken

1 tbsp. rosemary

1 tbsp. basil

1 tbsp. thyme

1/2 tsp. salt

1 tbsp. garlic, minced

1/2 tsp. pepper

1 tbsp. olive oil

1 lemon

Step-by-step Directions to Cook it:

1.   Mix all the dry ingredients, garlic, and oil in a bowl.

2.   Rub the mixture on the chicken and stuff some lemon inside the chicken.

3.   Roast the chicken for 40 minutes in a preheated PowerXL Air Fryer Grill.

Nutritional value per serving:

Calories: 127kcal, Protein: 26.3 g, Fat: 0.5 g.

284.Apple, Carrot, and Onion Stuffed Turkey

Prep time: 30 minutes | Cook time: 3 hours | Serves 12 to 14

1 (12-pound/5.4-kg) turkey, giblet removed, rinsed and pat dry

Seasoning:

¼ cup lemon pepper

2 tablespoons chopped fresh parsley

1 tablespoon celery salt

2 cloves garlic, minced

2 teaspoons ground black pepper

1 teaspoon sage

Stuffing:

1 medium onion, cut into 8 equal parts

1 carrot, sliced

1 apple, cored and cut into 8 thick slices

1.   Mix together the seasoning in a small bowl. Rub over the surface and inside of the turkey.

2.   Stuff the turkey with the onions, carrots, and apples. Using the rotisserie spit, push through the turkey and attach the rotisserie forks.

3.   If desired, place aluminum foil onto the drip pan. (It makes for easier clean-up!)

4.   Place the prepared turkey with rotisserie spit into the air fryer grill

5.   Select Toast, set temperature to 350ºF (180ºC), Rotate, and set time to 3 hours..

6.   When cooking is complete, the internal temperature should read at least 180 ºF (82 ºC). Remove the lamb leg using the rotisserie lift and, using hot pads or gloves, carefully remove the turkey from the spit.

7.   Server hot.

285.Spicy-Sweet Pork Tenderloin

Prep time: 20 minutes | Cook time: 25 minutes | Serves 2 to 3

1 pound (454 g) pork tenderloin

2 tablespoons Sriracha hot sauce

2 tablespoons honey

1½ teaspoons kosher salt

1.   Stir together the honey, Sriracha hot sauce, and salt in a bowl. Rub the sauce all over the pork tenderloin.

2.   Using the rotisserie spit, push through the pork tenderloin and attach the rotisserie forks.

3.   If desired, place aluminum foil onto the drip pan. (It makes for easier clean-up!)

4.   Place the prepared pork tenderloin with rotisserie spit into the air fryer grill.

5.   Select Air Fry, set temperature to 350ºF (180ºC), Rotate, and set time to 20 minutes.

6.   When cooking is complete, remove the pork tenderloin using the rotisserie lift and, using hot pads or gloves, carefully remove the chicken from the spit.

7.   Let rest for 5 minutes and serve.

286.Standing Rib Roast

This classic and comforting holiday meal is beyond any description.

Prep and Cooking time: 90 minutes | Serves: 8

Ingredients to Use:

5 lb. rib-eye meat

Salt & pepper

1 tbsp. thyme

1 tbsp. rosemary

1 stick unsalted butter

Step-by-step Directions to Cook it:

1.   Preheat the PowerXL Air Fryer Grill to 230ºC or 450ºF.

2.   Mix the butter and dry ingredients in a bowl.

3.   Rub the mixture on the rib and roast it for an hour in the preheated PowerXL Air Fryer Grill.

4.   Serve with fresh herbs on top.

Nutritional value per serving:

Calories: 185kcal, Protein: 52.0 g, Fat: 48 g.

287.Simple Air-Fried Beef Roast

Prep time: 5 minutes | Cook time: 38 minutes | Serves 6

2.5 pound (1.1 kg) beef roast

1 tablespoon olive oil

1 tablespoon Poultry seasoning

1.   Tie the beef roast and rub the olive oil all over the roast. Sprinkle with the seasoning.

2. Using the rotisserie spit, push through the beef roast and attach the rotisserie forks.
3. If desired, place aluminum foil onto the drip pan. (It makes for easier clean-up!)
4. Place the prepared chicken with rotisserie spit into the air fryer grill.
5. Select Air Fry. Set temperature to 360ºF (182ºC), and set time to 38 minutes for medium rare beef.
6. When cooking is complete, remove the beef roast using the rotisserie lift and, using hot pads or gloves, carefully remove the beef roast from the spit.
7. Let cool for 5 minutes before serving.

288.Air-Fried Lemony-Garlicky Chicken

Prep time: 10 minutes | Cook time: 45 minutes | Serves 4
3 pounds (1.4 kg) tied whole chicken
3 cloves garlic, halved
1 whole lemon, quartered
2 sprigs fresh rosemary whole
2 tablespoons olive oil
Chicken Rub:
½ teaspoon fresh ground pepper
½ teaspoon salt
1 teaspoon garlic powder
1 teaspoon dried oregano
1 teaspoon paprika
1 sprig rosemary (leaves only)
1. Mix together the rub ingredients in a small bowl. Set aside.
2. Place the chicken on a clean cutting board. Ensure the cavity of the chicken is clean. Stuff the chicken cavity with the garlic, lemon, and rosemary.
3. Tie your chicken with twine if needed. Pat the chicken dry.
4. Drizzle the olive oil all over and coat the entire chicken with a brush.
5. Shake the rub on the chicken and rub in until the chicken is covered.
6. Using the rotisserie spit, push through the chicken and attach the rotisserie forks.
7. If desired, place aluminum foil onto the drip pan. (It makes for easier clean-up!)
8. Place the prepared chicken with the rotisserie spit into the air fryer grill.
9. Select Air Fry, set the temperature to 375ºF (190ºC) . Set the time to 40 minutes. Check the temp in 5 minute increments after the 40 minutes.

10. At 40 minutes, check the temperature every 5 minutes until the chicken reaches 165ºF (74ºC) in the breast, or 165ºF (85ºC) in the thigh.
11. Once cooking is complete, remove the chicken using the rotisserie lift and, using hot pads or gloves, carefully remove the chicken from the spit.
12. Let the chicken sit, covered, for 5 to 10 minutes.
13. Slice and serve.

289.Roasted Vegetable Pasta

This hearty and easy pasta recipe will help you save your time and fill your tummy.
Prep and Cooking time: 30 minutes | Serves: 4
Ingredients to use:
10-ounce linguine pasta
1/2 cup cilantro, chopped
5 cherry tomatoes, chopped
1 zucchini, chopped
1/2 cup marinara sauce
Salt & pepper
1/2 cup parmesan cheese
2 tbsp. olive oil
Step-by-step Directions to Cook it:
1. **Preheat the PowerXL Air Fryer Grill to 1500C or 3000F.**
2. **Stir in the veggies, pasta, and spices in a bowl with some water.**
3. **Roast for 20 minutes.**
4. **Sprinkle parmesan cheese on top.**
Nutritional value per serving:
Calories: 179kcal, carbs: 40g, Protein: 6.3g, Fat: 1.5g

290.Air-Fried Whole Chicken

Prep time: 10 minutes | Cook time: 50 minutes | Serves 4
2 cups buttermilk
¼ cup olive oil
1 teaspoon garlic powder
1 tablespoon sea salt
1 whole chicken
Salt and pepper, to taste
1. In a large bag, place the buttermilk, oil, garlic powder, and sea salt and mix to combine.
2. Add the whole chicken and let marinate for 24 hours up to two days.
3. Remove the chicken and sprinkle with the salt and pepper.

4. Truss the chicken, removing the wings and ensuring the legs are tied closely together and the thighs are held in place.

5. Using the rotisserie spit, push through the chicken and attach the rotisserie forks.

6. If desired, place aluminum foil onto the drip pan. (It makes for easier clean-up!)

7. Place the prepared chicken with the rotisserie spit into the air fryer grill.

8. Select Air Fry, set the temperature to 380ºF (193ºC), Rotate, and set the time for 50 minutes.

9. When cooking is complete, the chicken should be dark brown and internal temperature should measure 165 degrees (measure at the meatiest part of the thigh).

10. Remove the chicken using the rotisserie lift and, using hot pads or gloves, carefully remove the chicken from the spit.

11. Let sit for 10 minutes before slicing and serving.

291.Honey-Glazed Ham

Prep time: 20 minutes | Cook time: 3 hours | Serves 6

1 (5-pound/2.3-kg) cooked boneless ham, pat dry
Glaze:
½ cup honey
2 teaspoons lemon juice
1 teaspoon ground cloves
1 teaspoon cinnamon
½ cup brown sugar

1. Using the rotisserie spit, push through the ham and attach the rotisserie forks.

2. If desired, place aluminum foil onto the drip pan. (It makes for easier clean-up!)

3. Place the prepared ham with rotisserie spit into the air fryer grill.

4. Select Toast, set temperature to 250ºF (121ºC), Rotate, and set time to 3 hours.

5. Meanwhile, combine the ingredients for the glaze in a small bowl. Stir to mix well.

6. When the ham has reached 145 ºF (63 ºC), brush the glaze mixture over all surfaces of the ham.

7. When cooking is complete, remove the ham using the rotisserie lift and, using hot pads or gloves, carefully remove the ham from the spit.

8. Let it rest for 10 minutes covered loosely with foil and then carve and serve.

292.Roasted Filet Mignon

Check out this classic steak recipe if you want to bring back the 90's vibe in your dinner table.

Prep and Cooking time: 30 minutes | Serves: 2
Ingredients to use:
10 ounces filet mignon
1 tbsp. Italian herbs, chopped
Salt & pepper
2 tbsp. olive oil
Step-by-step Directions to Cook it:
1. *Preheat the PowerXL Air Fryer Grill to 200ºC or 400ºF.*
2. *Mix all the seasonings and oil, and rub the mixture on the steak.*
3. *Roast it for 30 minutes.*
Nutritional value per serving:
Calories: 267kcal, Protein: 26g, Fat: 17g

293.Rotisserie Red Wine Lamb

Prep time: 25 minutes | Cook time: 1 hour 30 hours | Serves 6 to 8

1 (5-pound / 2.3-kg) leg of lamb, bone-in, fat trimmed, rinsed and drained
Marinade:
¼ cup dry red wine
1 large shallot, roughly chopped
4 garlic cloves, peeled and roughly chopped
5 large sage leaves
Juice of 1 lemon
2 teaspoons Worcestershire sauce
½ teaspoon allspice
¾ cup fresh mint leaves
3 tablespoons fresh rosemary
$^1/_3$ cup beef stock
½ teaspoon coriander powder
2 teaspoons brown sugar
½ teaspoon cayenne pepper
½ cup olive oil
2 teaspoons salt
1 teaspoon black pepper
Baste:
1 cup beef stock
¼ cup marinade mixture
Garnish: salt and black pepper

1. Combine the marinade ingredients in a large bowl. Stir to mix well. Remove ¼ cup of the marinade and set aside.

2.	Apply remaining marinade onto lamb leg. Place the lamb leg into a baking dish, cover and refrigerate for 1 to 2 hours.

3.	Combine the ingredients for the baste in a small bowl. Stir to mix well. Set aside until ready to use.

4.	Using the rotisserie spit, push through the lamb leg and attach the rotisserie forks.

5.	If desired, place aluminum foil onto the drip pan. (It makes for easier clean-up!)

6.	Place the prepared lamb leg with rotisserie spit into the air fryer grill.

7.	Select Toast, set temperature to 350ºF (180ºC), Rotate, and set time to 1 hour 30 minutes.

8.	After the first 30 minutes of cooking, apply the baste over the lamb leg for every 20 minutes.

9.	When cooking is complete, remove the lamb leg using the rotisserie lift and, using hot pads or gloves, carefully remove the lamb leg from the spit.

10.	Carve and serve.

294.Miso Glazed Salmon

Check out one of the quickest, easiest, and least messy ways to cook glazed salmon.

Prep and Cooking time: 15 minutes | Serves: 4

Ingredients to use:

 4 salmon filets

 1/4 cup miso

 1/3 cup sugar

 1 tsp. soy sauce

 1/3 cup sake

 2 tsp. vegetable oil

Step-by-step Directions to Cook it:

*1.	Whisk all the ingredients, except for filets, in a bowl.*

*2.	Marinate the filets with the mixture for 10 minutes.*

*3.	Preheat the PowerXL Air Fryer Grill to high and roast it for 5 minutes.*

Nutritional value per serving:

Calories: 331.8kcal, Carbs: 2gProtein: 34 g, Fat: 17.9 g.

295.Toasted Marinated Medium Rare Beef

Prep time: 15 minutes | Cook time: 1 hour 40 minutes | Serves 6 to 8

5 pounds (2.3 kg) eye round beef roast

2 onions, sliced

3 cups white wine

3 cloves garlic, minced

1 teaspoon chopped fresh rosemary

1 teaspoon celery seeds

1 teaspoon fresh thyme leaves

¾ cup olive oil

1 tablespoon coarse sea salt

1 tablespoon ground black pepper

1 teaspoon dried sage

2 tablespoons unsalted butter

1.	Place beef roast and onions in a large resealable bag.

2.	In a small bowl, combine the wine, garlic, rosemary, celery seeds, thyme leaves, oil, salt, pepper, and sage.

3.	Pour the marinade mixture over the beef roast and seal the bag. Refrigerate the roast for up to one day.

4.	Remove the beef roast from the marinade. Using the rotisserie spit, push through the beef roast and attach the rotisserie forks.

5.	If desired, place aluminum foil onto the drip pan. (It makes for easier clean-up!)

6.	Place the prepared lamb leg with rotisserie spit into the air fryer grill.

7.	Select Toast, set temperature to 400ºF (205ºC), Rotate, and set time to 1 hour 40 minutes. Baste the beef roast with marinade for every 30 minutes.

8.	When cooking is complete, remove the lamb leg using the rotisserie lift and, using hot pads or gloves, carefully remove the lamb leg from the spit.

9.	Remove the roast to a platter and allow the roast to rest for 10 minutes.

10.	 Slice thin and serve.

CHAPTER 15: BREAD & PIZZA

296. Pizza Toast

Try out the easiest recipe to satisfy your pizza cravings.

Prep and Cooking time: 5 minutes | Serves: 2

Ingredients to use:

4 slices bread.

1/2 cup grated mozzarella.

Pepperoni

1/2 tbsp. Italian herbs.

1/2 cup marinara sauce

Step-by-step Directions to Cook it:

1.   Spread marinara and grated cheese on the bread.

2.   Put pepperoni and sprinkle some oregano.

3.   Grill it in the preheated PowerXL Air Fryer Grill for 5 minutes.

Nutritional value per serving:

Calories: 175kcal, Carbs: 20g, Protein: 9g, Fat: 7g.

297. Baked Meatloaf

Here's an easy meatloaf recipe that is hard to resist.

Prep and Cooking time: 60 minutes | Serves: 4

Ingredients to use:

1 lb. ground beef

1 onion, chopped

1/2 cup tomato, diced

1 tbsp. Italian herbs

1 tbsp. paprika

1 egg

Salt & pepper

1/2 tbsp. garlic, minced

2 tbsp. olive oil

Step-by-step Directions to Cook it:

1.   Preheat the PowerXL Air Fryer Grill to 232°C or 450°F.

2.   Combine all the ingredients in a bowl.

3.   Grease a loaf pan with olive oil and put the mixture in it.

4.   Bake it for 40 minutes.

Nutritional value per serving:

Calories: 195kcal, Protein: 56g, Fat: 15g.

298. Strawberry Ricotta Toast

This hearty and insta-worthy breakfast will help you start the day right.

Prep and Cooking time: 10 minutes | Serves: 2

Ingredients to use:

2 slices of wheat bread

5 strawberries, chopped

100gm ricotta cheese

1 tbsp. ground cinnamon

2 eggs

2 tbsp. pistachios

Honey

Step-by-step Directions to Cook it:

1.   Whisk eggs with cinnamon in a bowl.

2.   Soak the bread slices in the egg mixture.

3.   Toast the bread in the preheated PowerXL Air Fryer Grill.

4.   Spread ricotta, strawberries, and pistachios on the freshly toasted bread.

5.   Drizzle some honey on top.

Nutritional value per serving:

Calories: 195kcal, Carbs: 10g, Protein: 15g, Fat: 4g.

299.Mediterranean Baked Fish

This delicate baked fish with a spicy kick will make your heart smile.

Prep and Cooking time: 20 minutes | Serves: 4

Ingredients to use:

4 white boneless fish fillets

1 large onion, diced

1 tomato, diced

1/2 tbsp. paprika

1/2 tbsp. cumin powder

1/2 tbsp. coriander powder

1 clove garlic, minced

3 tbsp. olive oil

1/3 cup lime juice

1/2 cup of water

Step-by-step Directions to Cook it:

1.   Mix all the ingredients and marinate the fillets for 10 minutes.

2.   Bake it in the PowerXL Air Fryer Grill for 10 minutes.

3.   Serve with fresh cilantro on top.

Nutritional value per serving:

Calories: 170kcal, Protein: 14g, Fat: 35g.

300.Baked Cinnamon Apple

Check out this baked apple recipe to satisfy your sweet tooth in a healthy way.

Prep and Cooking time: 10 minutes | Serves: 3

Ingredients to use:

3 apples, cut

1/2 tbsp. ground cinnamon

1/2 tbsp. vanilla

1 tbsp. brown sugar

Step-by-step Directions to Cook it:

1.   Preheat the PowerXL Air Fryer Grill to 120̥C or 250̥F.

2.   Coat the apples with cinnamon, sugar, and vanilla.

3.   Bake for 10 minutes. Serve with ice cream.

Nutritional value per serving:

Calories: 214kcal, Carbs: 36g, Protein: 0.4g, Fat: 0.9g.

CPSIA information can be obtained
at www.ICGtesting.com
Printed in the USA
LVHW060258150321
681534LV00036B/348